Eyesight and Imaging - Advances and New Perspectives

Edited by Alireza Ziaei and Michele Lanza

Published in London, United Kingdom

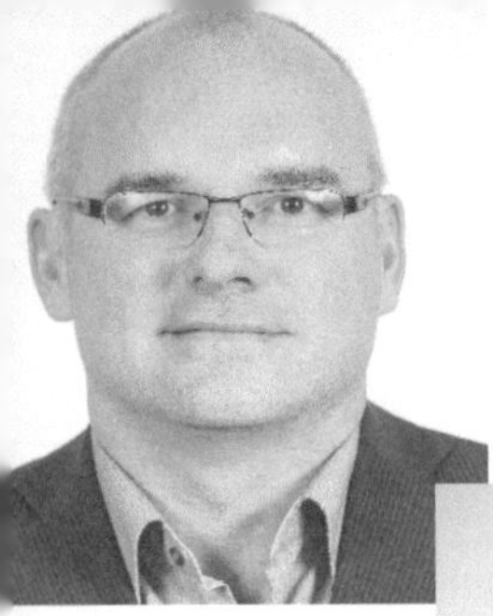
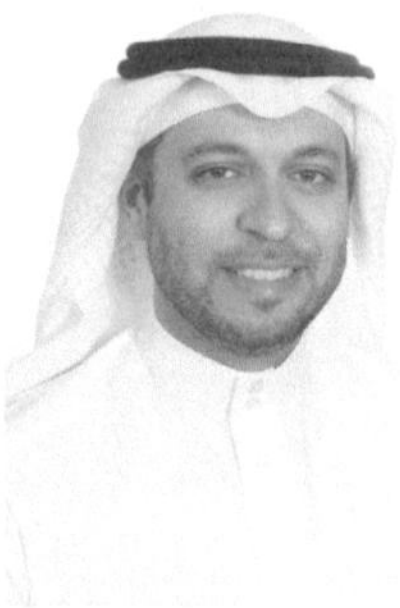
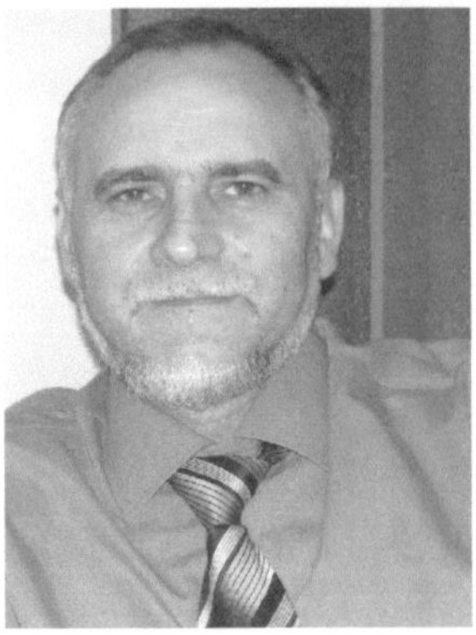
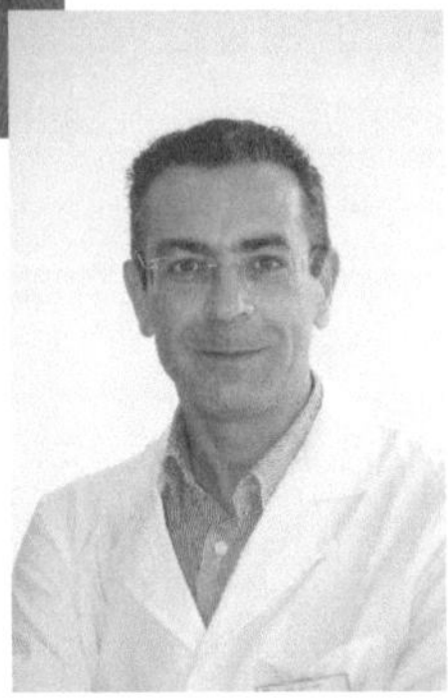
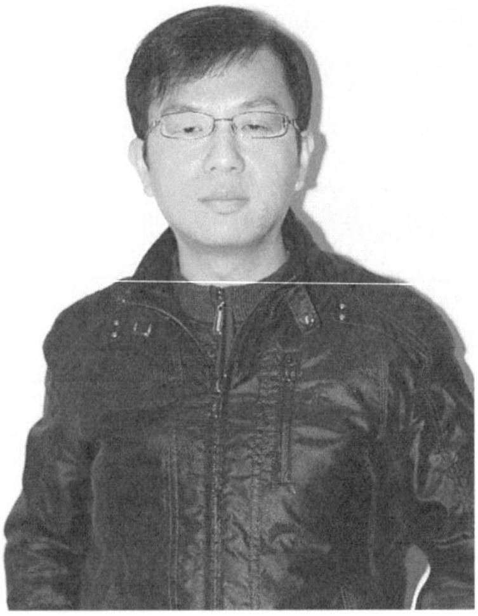
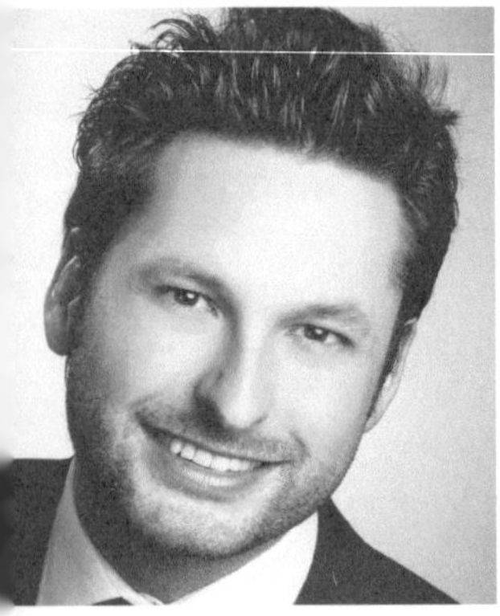
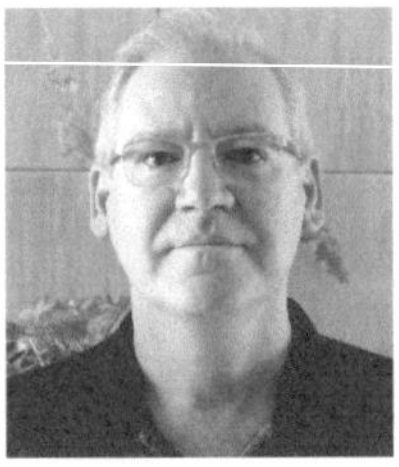

IntechOpen

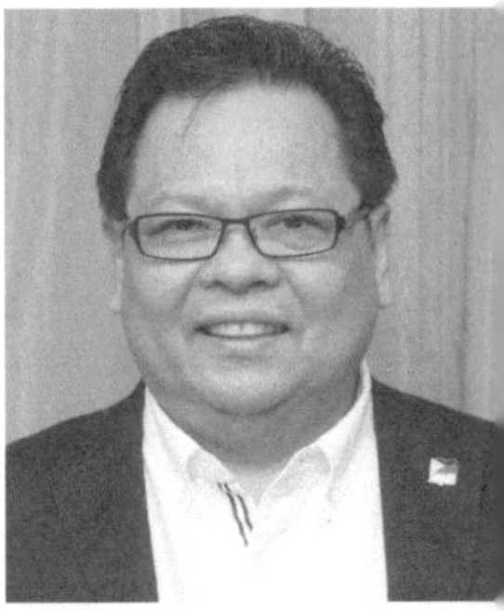
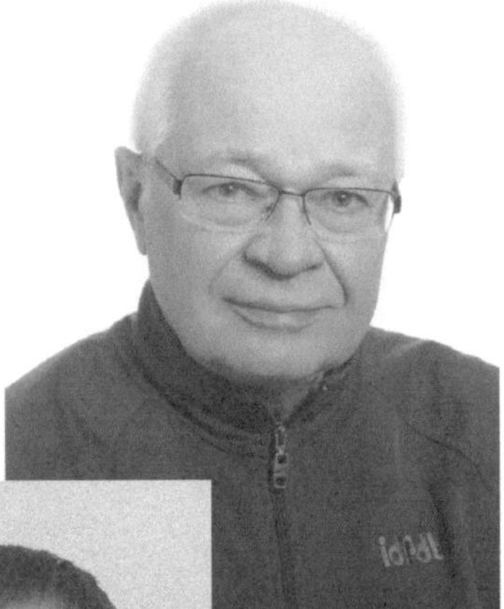
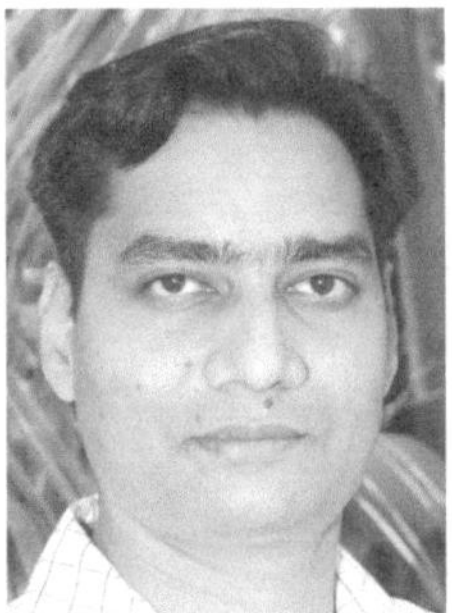
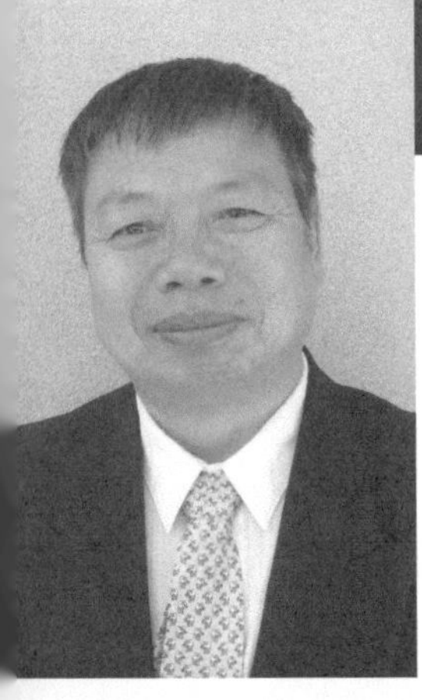
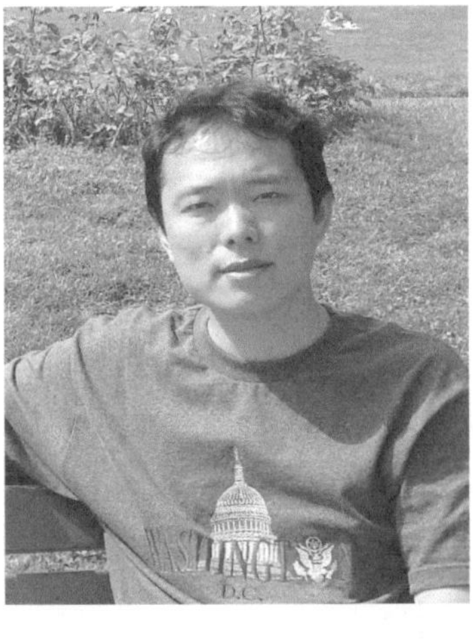
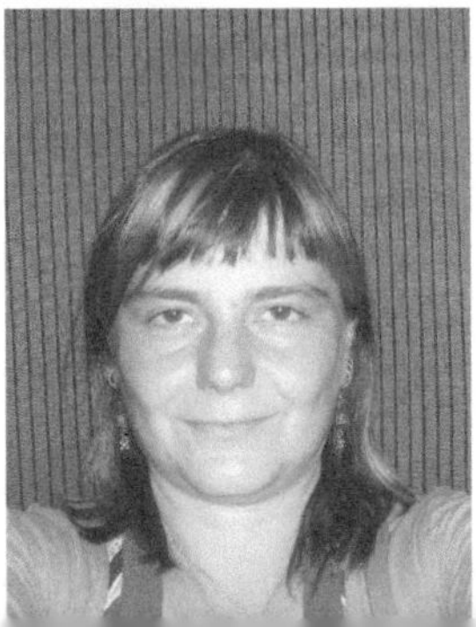

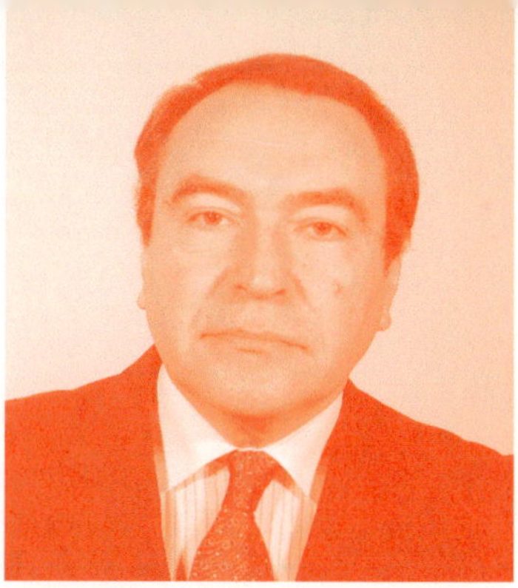
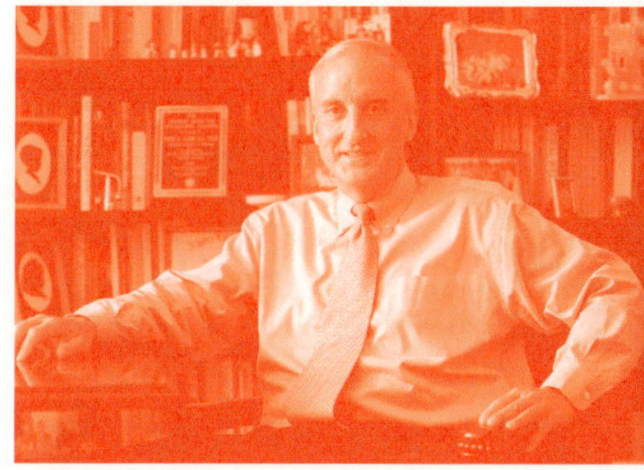
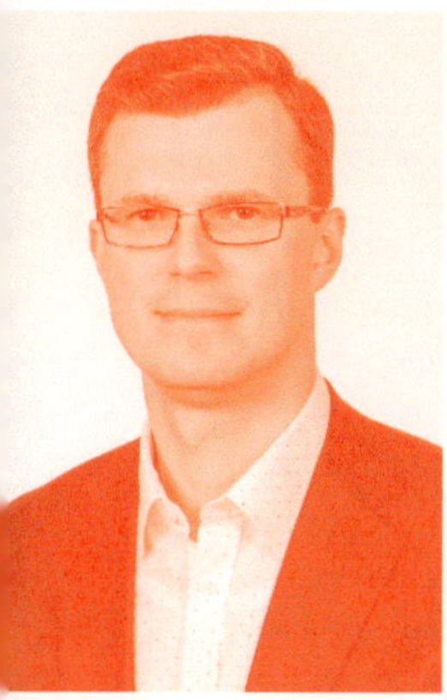
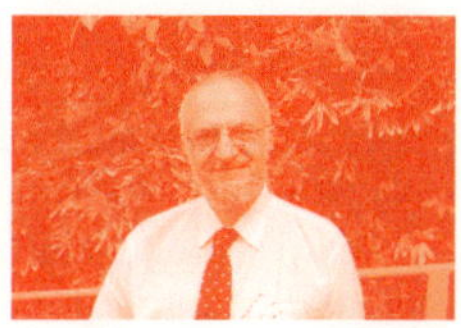
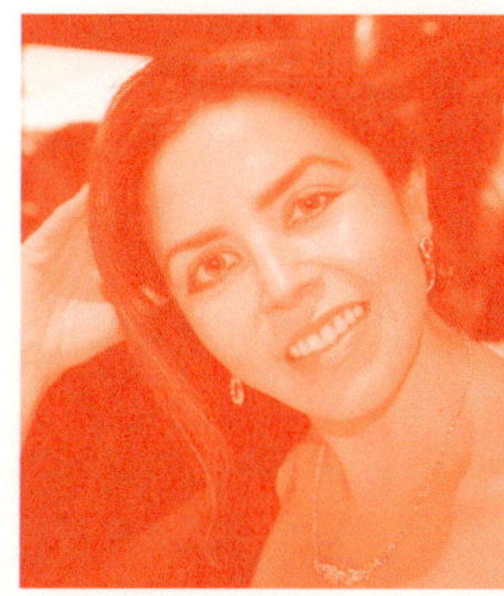

Supporting open minds since 2005

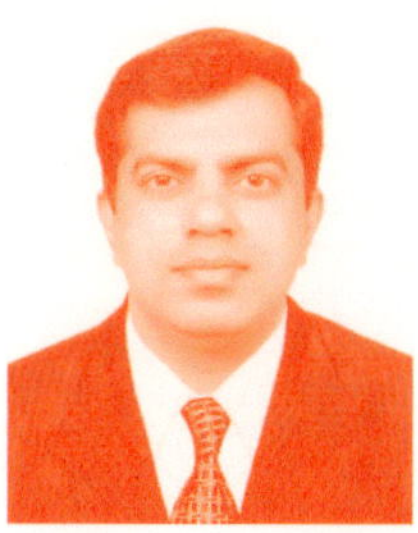
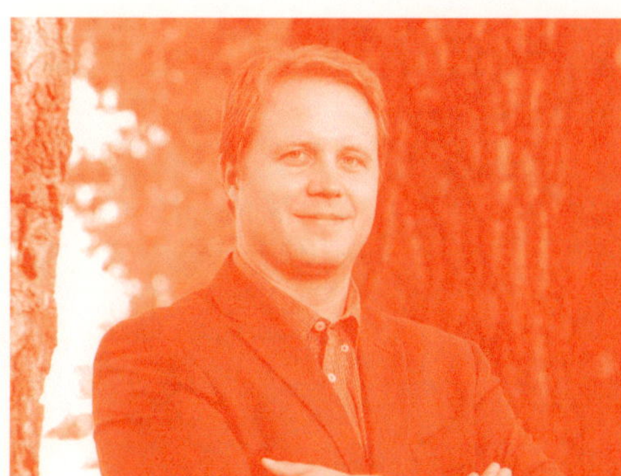
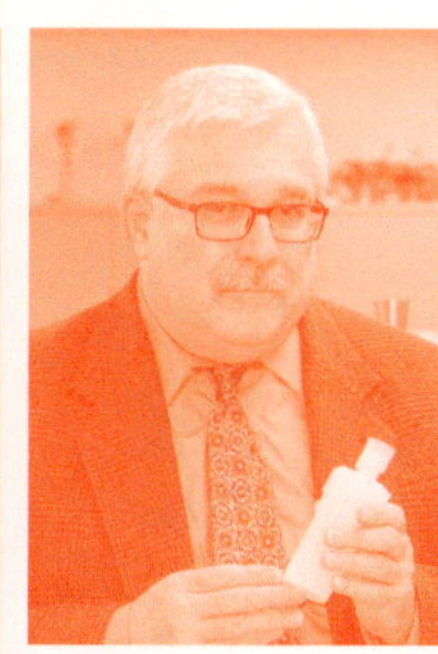
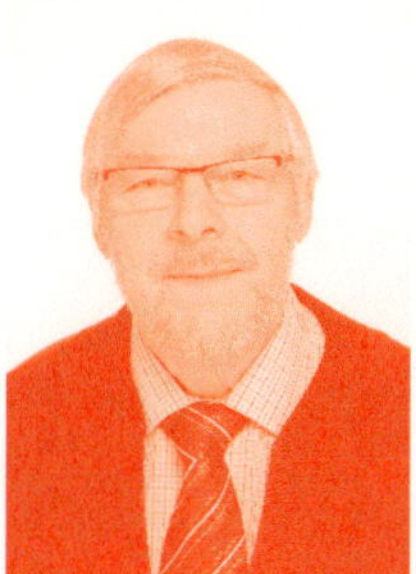
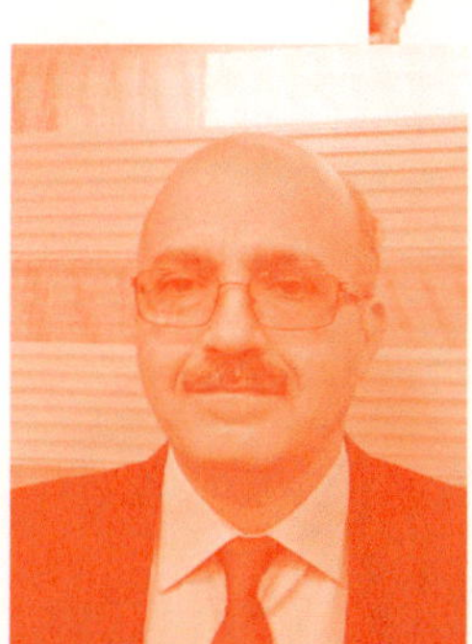
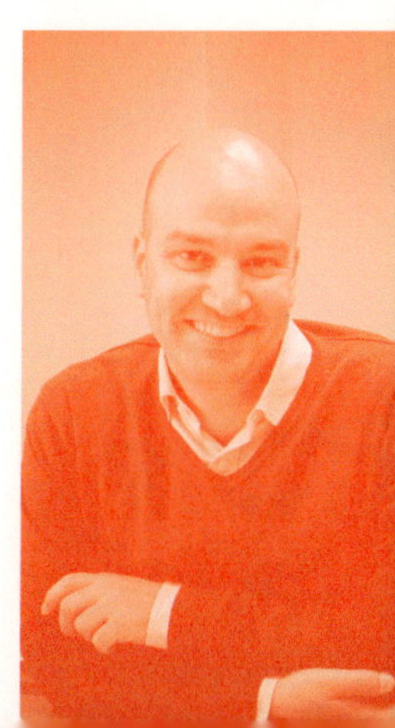
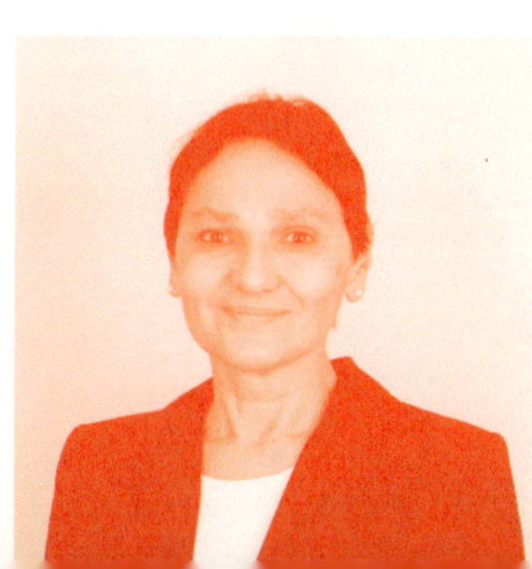

Eyesight and Imaging - Advances and New Perspectives
http://dx.doi.org/10.5772/intechopen.91289
Edited by Alireza Ziaei and Michele Lanza

Contributors
Dominique Monnet, Rung-Sheng Chen, Praveen Subudhi, Sweta Patro, Nageswar Rao Subudhi, Vatookarn Roongpoovapatr, Puwat Charukamnoetkanok, Mohamed Abou Shousha, Ersin Muhafiz, Clemence Bonnet, Saba Al-Hashimi, Antoine P. Brézin

First published in London, United Kingdom, 2021 by IntechOpen
IntechOpen is the global imprint of INTECHOPEN LIMITED, registered in England and Wales, registration number: 11086078, 5 Princes Gate Court, London, SW7 2QJ, United Kingdom
Printed in Croatia

British Library Cataloguing-in-Publication Data
A catalogue record for this book is available from the British Library

Additional hard and PDF copies can be obtained from orders@intechopen.com

Eyesight and Imaging - Advances and New Perspectives
Edited by Alireza Ziaei and Michele Lanza
p. cm.
Print ISBN 978-1-83880-955-3
Online ISBN 978-1-83880-956-0
eBook (PDF) ISBN 978-1-83880-957-7

Meet the editors

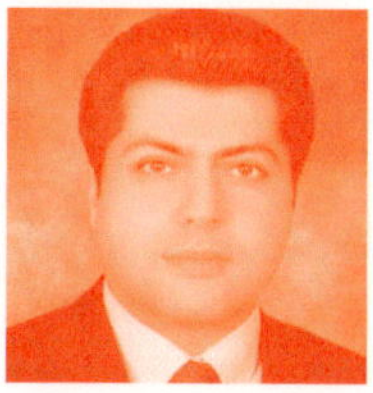

Dr. Alireza Ziaei, MD, is a physician-scientist at Harvard Medical School, Boston, USA. He is a recipient of numerous awards, including the National Excellent Researcher Award, National Young Investigator Award, and Science Excellence Prize. His main areas of interest are medical image processing and analysis, molecular basis and pathology pathways of ophthalmic disease, radiological detection, and image-guided therapy. He has considerable experience in biomedical research at Schepens Eye Research Institute, Massachusetts Eye and Ear, with a focus on corneal and ocular surface diseases, and at National Center for Image-Guided Therapy, Brain Tumor Consortium, and BCH Neuroimaging Center on radiological cancer detection at Harvard BWH/BCH hospitals. Dr. Ziaei's seminal work has been recognized several times. He has published and presented numerous articles in highly ranked peer-reviewed journals and conferences worldwide. Dr. Ziaei has been a scientific member of the Association for Research in Vision and Ophthalmology (ARV), American Academy of Ophthalmology (AAO), International Society for Magnetic Resonance in Medicine (ISMRM), Radiological Society of North America (RSNA), International Society for Brain Mapping and Therapeutics (ISBMT), Tear Film and Ocular Surface Society (TFOS), and Massachusetts Medical Society (MMS). He serves as an executive editor, editorial board member, and scientific reviewer of reputed journals and scientific societies, including Nature International Journal of Science, Journal of Magnetic Resonance Imaging, Abdominal Radiology, Investigative Ophthalmology & Visual Science (IOVS), American Journal of Ophthalmology (AJO), Journal of Clinical & Experimental Ophthalmology, and Journal of Cell Biology.

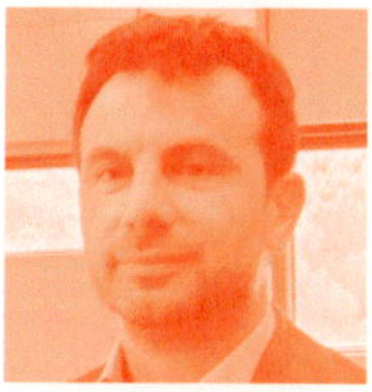

Michele Lanza is Associate Professor of Ophthalmology at Università della Campania, Luigi Vanvitelli, Napoli, Italy. His fields of interest are anterior segment disease, keratoconus, glaucoma, corneal dystrophies, and cataracts. His research topics include intraocular lens power calculation, eye modification induced by refractive surgery, glaucoma progression, and validation of new diagnostic devices in ophthalmology. He has published more than 100 papers in international and Italian scientific journals, more than 60 in journals with impact factors, and chapters in international and Italian books. He has also edited two international books and authored more than 150 communications or posters for the most important international and Italian ophthalmology conferences.

Contents

Preface

Imagination is the key to any discovery, and its presence in science to improve eyesight is no exception. The eyes are our windows to the brain and vision is the ability to interpret and understand the information that comes in through the eyes. The visual system utilizes brain pathways to process and understand what the eyes sense. The dynamic process of vision is to identify, interpret, and understand what the eyes see. An image is a sight that has been recreated and an appearance detached from the place and time in which it first appeared.

Blindness is an important symptom of many eye disorders. The estimated global cost of vision loss today is US$3 trillion. Science and research have always been crucial to furthering our understanding of ophthalmic conditions and their treatment and prevention. Ophthalmology research has resulted in major advancements in medical science and ophthalmic practice. Discoveries made in various fields including genetics, immunology, and ocular biology have reshaped the foundations of ophthalmology and formed many new paradigms for the repair, regeneration, and rehabilitation of countless disorders. Scientific achievements in ophthalmology have produced fundamental insights and opened up possibilities for improving human health. A major challenge for the next decade will be to translate these advances into identifying the design and testing of novel approaches for disease treatments.

This book provides readers with a comprehensive overview of the latest and most advanced findings in several aspects of ophthalmic pathology, treatment, and surgical strategies, as well as in vision sciences and perception. Chapters cover such topics as acute hydrops, cataract treatments, keratoconus, surgical/non-surgical treatments in vision rehabilitation, and geometric analysis of ophthalmic lens.
I thank all the contributors for their kind efforts in the preparation of this book.

Alireza Ziaei, MD
Harvard Medical School BCH,
Boston, USA

Michele Lanza
University of Campania "Luigi Vanvitelli",
Italy

Chapter 1

Acute Hydrops and Its Management

Praveen Subudhi, Sweta Patro and Nageswar Rao Subudhi

Abstract

Acute hydrops is a well-known complication of keratoconus. It usually manifests as sudden onset loss of vision. Mostly presents in the pubertal age group. Allergic conjunctivitis associated with eye rubbing is the most substantial risk factor. Primary pathology being stromal lysis, which triggers the progression of cone, causing an undue stretch on Descemet Membrane, eventually resulting in its splitting and stromal imbibition of aqueous through these ruptures. Clinical signs are circumcillary congestion and thick/edematous cornea with obscuration of the anterior segment. Conservative therapy delays wound healing; hence early surgical intervention is recommended globally for faster resolution of stromal edema. Long-standing corneal edema mounts to corneal perforation and neovascularisation of cornea. Compressive suture, non expansile intracameral gas injection, Deep anterior lamellar keratoplasty, and mini Descemet membrane keratoplasty are various management modalities reported in literature. Acute hydrops could be well prevented with early identification of progressive keratoconus and halting its progression.

Keywords: acute hydrops, keratoconus, compressive sutures, intracameral gas, ocular allergy

1. Introduction

1.1 Epidemiology

Acute hydrops is a well-known complication of progressive keratoconus. It has also been reported in other noninflammatory ectatic disorders such as pellucid marginal degeneration and keratoglobus. The incidence of acute hydrops is minimal but varies according to race. A 2011 UK census reported higher number of cases among the South Asian and Black ethnic groups, compared with that in the general population. The reported incidence rates among the white, South Asian, and black population are 0.07/100,000, 0.32 /100,000, and 0.37/100,000, respectively [1]. According to numerous studies, the trend in acute hydrops Incidence among patients with keratoconus has been shown to be decreasing; Tuft et al. and Amsler M et al. reported the prevalence of acute hydrops as 2.6% and 2.8%, respectively [2, 3]. Acute hydrops can occur at any age but is commonly reported in individuals aged between 20 and 30 years, whereas the broad age range is 10 to 47 years. It has a significant gender disparity; men are more susceptible to this condition compared with women, with a ratio of 1.2:1 according to the Auckland Keratoconus Study [4], 3:1 according to a UK prospective study [1], and 2.9:1 according to an American study [5].

2. Predisposing factors

Ocular allergy is frequently associated with keratoconus ranging from 7 to 35% [6–9]. Bawazeer et al. in a case control study demonstrated a positive correlation between keratoconus and atopy [10]. Any form of ocular allergy instigates itching, foreign body sensation, and eye rubbing [11]. This triggers a corneal intrastromal inflammation because of the increased levels of histamine, tumor necrosis factor-alpha, and interleukins [12]. It coaxes to stromal lysis and corneal thinning because of the increased levels of lysosomal and proteolytic enzymes with a simultaneous reduction in the levels of protease inhibitors [12]. This vicious cycle of inflammation and stromal lysis is exacerbated by recurrent eye rubbing [13], and the stable keratoconus eventually becomes progressive which increases the risk of acute hydrops [14].

A history of having worn the contact lenses, specially the rigid gas permeable lens, is also considered an important risk factor for acute hydrops [15]. Contact lens usage triggers ocular inflammation because of hypoxia of the corneal surface [16]. A study showed that the level of inflammatory markers present in the tear film increases after the use of contact lens [17]. This inflammation initiates the progression of keratoconus that eventually leads to acute hydrops [18].

A trivial ocular trauma plays a significant role in the rupturing of already stressed-out descemet membrane (DM) [19]. Advanced keratoconus, eccentric cone, and poor visual acuity are other important risk factors for acute hydrops in patients with keratoconus. Down syndrome increases the risk of keratoconus progression, thereby increasing the risk of acute hydrops [20]. Retinitis pigmentosa, Leber Congenital Amaurosis (LCA), floppy eye lid syndrome, and Ehler-Danlos syndrome are other risk factors for progressive keratoconus, which are followed by the incident of hydrops [21–24]. Pregnancy and lactation are also the critical but temporary risk factors [25]. However, a positive family history has been reported to have a negative correlation with the acute hydrops incidence [26].

3. Corneal topography and acute hydrops

Corneal topography plays a critical role in identifying patients with keratoconus progression [27]. Various parameters are available in pentacam that must be reinvestigated after every 3 month to accurately diagnose the progression; parameters, namely, maximum keratometry, minimum pachymetry, pachymetric progression index, elevation indices of corneal front and back surfaces, anterior radius of curvature taken 3 mm surrounding the thinnest pachymetry, posterior radius of curvature taken 3 mm surrounding the thinnest pachymetry, and deviation index, must be scrutinized during every visit. Any evidence of progression should be intervened to prevent or halt the deterioration to eventually decrease the risk of acute hydrops incidence [28].

4. Pathophysiology

The progression of keratoconus initiates because of stretching of the DM that is adhered strongly to the periphery, which leads to circumferential stretching of the membrane and increased risk of its rupture [29, 30]. If the stretching extends beyond a limit, the membrane tends to rupture at the center, which leads to the seepage of aqueous fluid into the stroma and thereby causes acute hydrops [31].

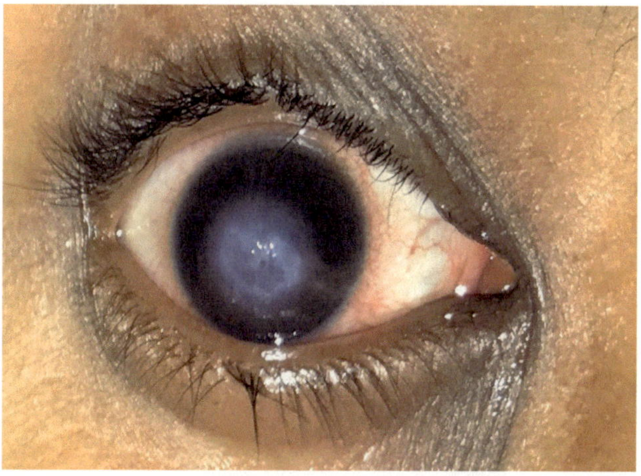

Figure 1.
Showing a case of acute hydrops.

5. Clinical examination and manifestations

Acute hydrops initiates with a sudden onset of poor vision and discoloration of the cornea [32]. The disease is confined to the central and paracentral regions and rarely manifests in the peripheral region in case of coexistent pellucid marginal degeneration [33]. In addition to a defective vision, pain and redness are the typical symptoms of this disease [34]. The patients exhibit a definite history of persisting poor vision since childhood and experience progressive vision loss [35]. History of spectacle use should be investigated by reviewing the old optical prescriptions or old spectacles. Past history of high astigmatism, oblique axis and poor best corrected visual acuity are considered as corroborative clinical signs of acute hydrops following progressive keratoconus. Meticulous medical history of ocular allergy, atopic dermatitis, contact lens usage, eye rubbing, and ocular trauma should be documented [36]. Contact lens history, with emphasis on the type, duration of usage, overnight usage while sleeping, and expiry date of the contact lens, is also considered essential [37]. Ocular trauma history, with emphasis on the blunt trauma not withstanding its impact or severity, should also be documented (**Figure 1**) [38].

Examination using a diffused torchlight reveals a whitish lesion over the central or paracentral regions with intense photophobia (**Figure 1**). Conjunctiva shows a sign of circumciliary congestion, and palpebral conjunctiva may be congested depending upon the presence of allergic conjunctivitis. In the absence of oculi allergy, eyes are less susceptible to palpebral congestion. The iris or anterior segment is not visible in case of central hydrops but in cases of paracentral hydrops, the anterior segment is clearly visible through the clear cornea [35].

Slit lamp examination with an oblique slit shows an abnormally thick cornea with clefts in the intrastromal area and Obscuration of Descemet Membrane (DM) due to the blockage of light rays by the edematous cornea [39, 40].

6. Grading of acute hydrops

Acute hydrops can be graded depending on the corneal region involved. Corneal edema can be graded by drawing an imaginary circle around the cornea [41].

Grade 1: Involves 3-mm diameter of cornea.
Grade 2: Between 3- and 5-mm diameter of cornea.
Grade 3: More than 5 m-diameter of cornea.

7. Investigations

Though acute hydrops is mostly diagnosed clinically, anterior segment OCT (ASOCT) can be performed to assess the severity and pattern of the resolution (**Figure 2**), [42]. ASOCT manifests as hypo reflective areas in the presence of fluid, hyper-reflective areas in the presence of fibrous tissues. In the early phase of corneal edema, epithelial micro cysts with pseudocysts formation in the intrastromal area are

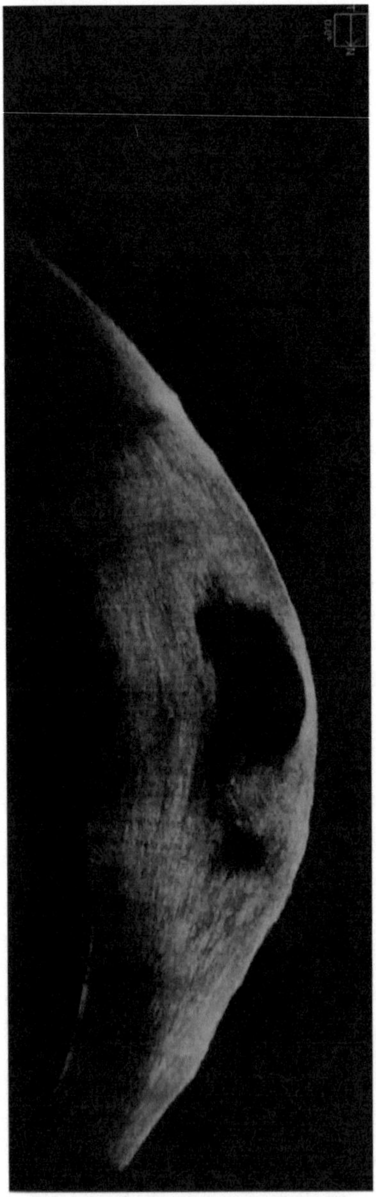

Figure 2.
ASOCT showing corneal edema, clefts and cysts (courtesy-Dr.Sridevi Gunda).

witnessed as hyporeflective areas [43]. Pseudocysts develop due to fluid accumulation in the intrastromal spaces separating the stromal lamellae because of the sudden egress of the fluid. The word "pseudocyst" was coined because the cyst wall formation does not involve epithelium. These pseudocysts are initially small in size and multiple in number but eventually they fuse to become a large cyst [44]. Sometimes, the fluid reaches the anterior stroma leading to bullous swelling of the corneal surface, referred as "epitheliocoele" in literature [45]. High-resolution ASOCT can demonstrate a breach in the continuity of the DM and stromal access to the aqueous humor [46]. ASOCT can also demonstrate a slow healing process of polygonal defects in the DM that is caused by its rupture. Healing of DM takes place slowly than that of the corneal epithelium. Hence, decrease in the size of DM defect can be witnessed after a week, and in the due course, the corneal edema which is seen as hypo-reflective/dark areas gets reduced eventually allowing the visibility of hyper-reflective shadows in the sub epithelial area marks the healing of acute hydrops [46].

Confocal microscopy is a new modality in the investigation process; though it is more useful for academic purpose, it gives an insight into the pathology of the disease [47]. Confocal microscope acts like an in vivo electron microscope; hence, the technique is termed as in vivo confocal microscopy (IVCM). It analyses the anterior and middle parts of the cornea. Bullae are seen in the superficial and wing layers of the corneal epithelium. Stromal area shows hyper-reflective band-shaped structures in the anterior stroma, and microfilms are seen in the mid and anterior stroma. Hyper-reflective cells are seen in the anterior stroma and epithelium, which are presumed to be inflammatory cells [48].

8. Complications

Acute hydrops commonly resolves spontaneously over a period of 4–8 weeks; however, it can be delayed because of large DM deficit or poor functionality of the corneal endothelial cells [49].

The risk of corneal perforation in cases of extreme penetration of fluid into the anterior stromal space is also present, which results in the formation of the epithelial bullae [50]. Any trivial trauma or ocular rubbing causes the rupture of the bullae, which may lead to shallowing of an anterior chamber and the formation of an anterior synechiae. Upon healing, it forms a dense vascularized corneal scar with extremely poor prognosis [51].

Corneal vascularization can be accentuated with a delay in the process of corneal edema reduction. Long-term cornea edema is associated with a risk of the release of vascular endothelial growth factors that induces corneal vasculogenesis from the peripheral corneal vessels, eventually leading to the formation of a vascularized corneal scar [51].

Bullous rupture of the corneal surface exposes raw stroma to the tear film and ocular commensals. Poor hygienic practices may lead to infectious keratitis [52]. Mostly bacterial keratitis has been reported; however, fungal keratitis has also been reported in the tropical countries. In developing countries such as India, the use of over-the-counter topical corticosteroids without clinical consultation is rampant that has led to the development of debilitating infectious keratitis [53].

9. Differential diagnosis

Penetrating ocular trauma may mimic acute hydrops; however, it has a recent background history of trauma and entry wound [54].

Calotropis keratitis commonly seen in the Indian subcontinent seen after accidental fall of whitish fluid while plucking the flower of the plant [55]. It may be localized or diffused and mostly presents as emergency having a perfectly normal vision before the fall. Upon slit lamp examination, a typical DM folds with the corneal edema are visible, and no breach in the continuity of DM is detected.

Post-herpetic endothelial dysfunctions are seen typically after an episode of herpetic keratitis or most likely after herpes zoster ophthalmicus. Clinically, it is seen as the localized corneal edema with pigment dusting of the endothelium and the presence of sectoral iris atrophy in case of herpes zoster [56, 57].

CMV keratitis is another rarely seen condition of the cornea that can be considered for the differential diagnosis of acute hydrops, and it typically manifests as a focal corneal edema and appears as a coin-shaped lesion [58].

Nuclear fragment retention after cataract surgery is a rare but a significant differential diagnosis, which manifests as on- and off-focal corneal edema mostly in the inferior quadrant. A careful clinical examination of an anterior segment reveals the presence of nuclear fragments and a positive history of recurrent anterior uveitis [59].

Bullous keratopathy due to Fuchs endothelial corneal dystrophy can be ruled out by seeing the other eye [60].

10. Medical management

Medical management is mostly supportive and not definitive [61]. Pressure bandages may be helpful in reducing the corneal edema; however, it increases the risk of bullous rupture with vascularized corneal scar. A study reported that the use of bandage contact lens decreases the corneal edema but increases the corneal hypoxia, which delays the process of corneal healing and causes dense scar [62]. Topical hypertonic saline (5%) eye drops are used to treat acute corneal edema to enhance dryness of the cornea, and these eye drops work by pulling the water out of the cornea thorough an osmotic pattern. Additionally, the risk of epithelial breakage is decreased, which in turn decreases the risk of secondary infection. However, the patients experience a severe burning sensation and discomfort after using the eye drop. Hence, the efficacy of these eye drops is questionable. Topical corticosteroid eye drops can be used to decrease the inflammation and improve the endothelial functioning. These may also decrease the corneal neovascularization and symptomatic ocular discomfort. However, the topical corticosteroid eye drop usage is associated with an increased risk of steroid-induced glaucoma, cataract, and infectious keratitis over the ruptured bullae. Hence, it should be used cautiously with close follow-ups [61].

11. Surgical management

Various modalities of surgical management have been mentioned in literature to augment the process of corneal healing. All the methods mentioned in literature are equally efficient, providing a favorable visual outcome and preventing the formation of the corneal vascularization.

Primary surgical intention for acute hydrops is not to restore or confer a normal vision but hasten the resolution of corneal edema which eventually leads to a non-vascularised scar improving the prognosis for corneal transplantation.

Surgical modalities are as follows:

- Compressive sutures (**Figures 3** and **4**)
- Intracameral gas
- Combination of compressive sutures and intracameral gas (**Figure 5**)
- Deep anterior lamellar keratoplasty (DALK)
- Mini Descemet membrane endothelial keratoplasty (mini-DMEK)

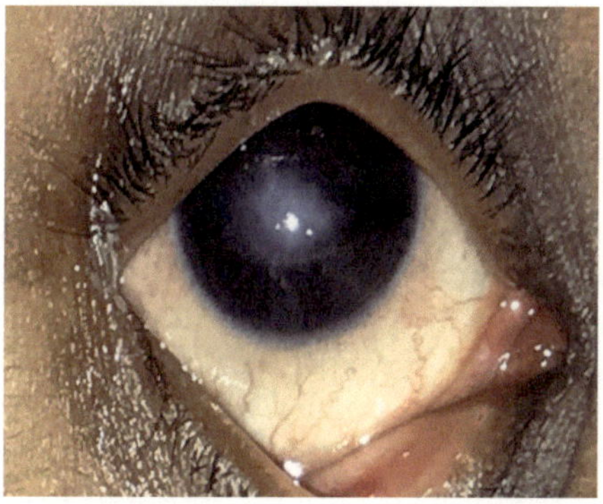

Figure 3.
Showing resolution of corneal edema after application of compressive sutures.

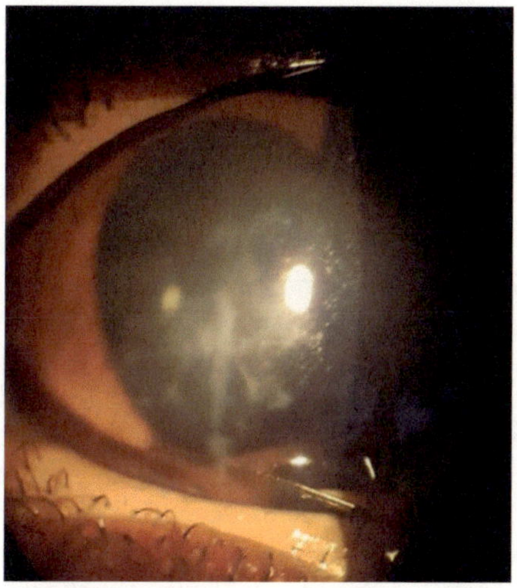

Figure 4.
Complete resolution of corneal edema with clear visualization of anterior segment structures.

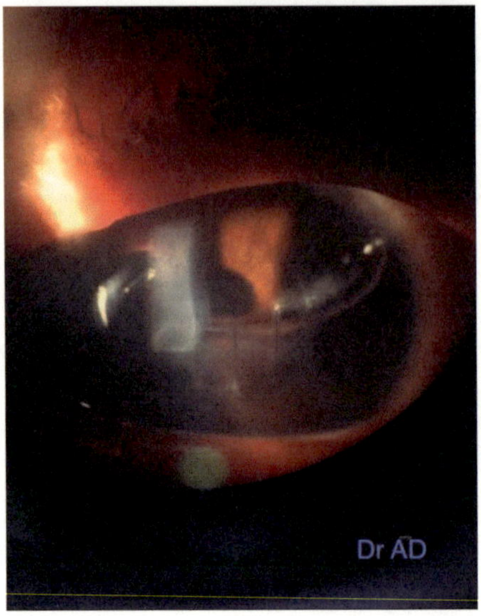

Figure 5.
Combination of compressive sutures with intracameral SF6 gas (Dr.Devi Aiswarya Das).

12. Intracameral gas

It is considered a treatment of choice for acute hydrops. Gas or air in an anterior chamber has 2 distinct advantages: first, it aids in the unrolling of the DM, and second, it provides compression of the DM to the swollen stroma [63, 64]. An injection of air was tried but it got absorbed in 3 days without giving enough tamponade to the DM. Hence, a nonexpansile mixture of the expansile gas with air is used to maintain the tamponade effect for a minimum period of 10 days. Sulfur hexafluoride (SF6) and perfluoropropane (C3F8) are commonly used by the corneal surgeons worldwide to produce a prolonged tamponade effect. SF6 (0.1 mL, 20%) was used by Panda et al. in their study of 9 cases that showed only marginal improvement in 3 cases and the remaining 6 cases required reintroduction of the gas twice or more for complete resolution of the corneal edema [63]. Basu et al. performed a comparative study on patients with acute hydrops [64]. One arm of the patients was treated with 14% nonexpansile perfluoropropane (C3F8), wheras the other arm was treated with conventional medical therapy. A faster resolution of the corneal edema was observed in the eyes of patients who were surgically treated, and the improvement was statistically significant. All the patients were advised to rest in a supine position for a period of 10 days to augment the tamponade effect. Histopathological studies on resolved hydrops have confirmed that DM adherence to the stroma is superior with intracameral gas compared with that without any treatment. All authors in the referred studies have recommended the continuation of conventional medical therapy of hypertonic saline eye drops, corticosteroids, and antiglaucoma drugs in the postoperative period. Nevertheless, acute hydrops treated using intracameral gas poses a high risk of pupillary block glaucoma, Urrets-Zavala syndrome, stromal cleft, and accidental seepage of air bubbles into the cornea stroma resembles a 'fish egg' in appearance in a slit lamp experiment. Hence, an inferior surgical iridectomy is recommended to prevent any instances of acute congestive glaucoma. Moreover, the intracameral gas should be introduced along the iris plane and in a single bubble because faulty introduction of the gas may lead to the bursting of the bubble into multiple bubbles that will nullify the tamponade effect and cause accidental damage to the corneal endothelium and seepage of the bubbles into the stroma.

13. Compressive sutures

Full-thickness corneal sutures involving the edematous part of the cornea have facilitated decrease in the corneal edema [30]. Here a 10–0 nylon suture is used to tamponade the Descemet membrane to corneal stroma. Initially a small paracentesis is created at the limbus of cornea followed by injection of intracameral pilocarpine to constrict the pupil. Viscoelastics are injected into the anterior chamber next to protect iris and crystalline lens. A 10–0 nylon suture is introduced at the junction of edematous and non-edematous cornea, the curved needle once enters the anterior chamber is taken out from the farthest end of the needle with a distance equivalent to the length of the needle and is tied over the corneal surface. The knot of a suture is buried into the cornea. Multiple sutures can be applied depending on the extent of the edema. The basic purpose of compressive sutures is not to oppose the torn DM ends but just to provide a support to the DM by bringing it near to the stroma. Once DM is opposed to the stromal endothelial cells, it starts pumping out a fluid from the stroma by active filtration and thereby helps in faster resolution of the corneal edema. Subudhi et al. demonstrated an excellent visual outcome associated with the use of compressive sutures alone in the management of acute hydrops; visual acuity of the patient improved from hand movements to 6/24 by the end of 2 months with a minimal scar at the center and no evidence of any corneal vascularization. Compressive sutures can be applied in a linear manner in case of small hydrops, but if hydrops is large enough to cover nearly all portions of the cornea, then a rectangular pattern involving all the quadrants can be applied. Pads and bandages can be given for a period of 24 hours to prevent any egress of fluid from the anterior chamber and its shallowing. Intracameral antibiotics can be given as prophylactic measures. These sutures stay for a period of 2 to 3 weeks; loosening of the sutures causes loss in the tamponade effect and should be removed in an operating room under strict aseptic precautions. Adverse effects observed are the shallow anterior chamber on Post-Operative Day 1; however, they got resolved in 24 hours without any further intervention. Nonetheless, these patients were advised to perform their routine activity after 5 days of rest. No patients were advised to have a mandatory supine position as in the treatment with intracameral gas injection.

14. Combination of intracameral gas and compressive sutures

In a view of complications associated with the single use of the intracameral gas or compressive sutures, Rajaraman and associates suggested a combination of compressive sutures and intracameral gas to incorporate the advantages of both the procedures [64]. Compressive sutures prevent the seepage of air bubbles into the intrastromal space and the intracameral gas prevents the shallowing of the anterior chamber in an immediate postoperative period following the application of the full-thickness compressive sutures.

15. Anterior chamber paracenetesis with thermokeratoplasty

In this procedure paracentesis is done to reduce the intraocular pressure so that the tension of aqueous humor over Descemet membrane is eliminated subsequently thermokeratoplasty is done to induce stromal contraction thus outward expansion of stroma due to edematous cornea is reduced. Hence eventually hastening the resolution of acute hydrops [65].

16. DALK

Anterior lamellar keratoplasty [66] in the pretext of acute hydrops is a difficult and complex procedure. Susan et al. recommended a modified DALK method for the treatment of acute hydrops. Small aliquots of air are injected into the stroma, immediately above the predescemeticdua layer and away from the site of the descemet rupture. Subsequently, a lamellar dissection with the help of a blunt crescent is performed carefully in the peripheral cornea, while avoiding the site of the DM tear initially, and then dissected at the center by slowly peeling the stroma. A donor cornea of the same size or 0.25 mm oversize is placed over the raw recipient corneal surface and anchored with the help of twelve or sixteen 10–0 nylon sutures. This averts the two-step procedure, which is normally adopted for acute hydrops, and thus, the visual rehabilitation is gained with a single procedure. However, because of edematous cornea, the risk of augmentation of the DM tear is increased and locating a correct plane for dissection becomes difficult for the surgeons. Therefore, surgeons are advised to become well-versed with anterior lamellar keratoplasty before advocating this procedure.

17. Mini-DMEK

It is another [67] procedure described in literature. Bachmann and associates described a novel technique of replacing the torn DM with a well-circumscribed donor DM. In this technique, the peripheral torn DM is trimmed and stripped up to the center of the cornea. But the crux of the matter here is that all the maneuvers are performed with an intraoperative OCT-enabled microscope. The donor DM is prepared depending on the defect and is introduced into the anterior chamber with the help of the lens cartridge. Rolled DM enters into the anterior chamber and is unrolled with the help of 2 Sinskey hooks by pressing one end and ironing the other end of corneal lenticule over the anterior corneal surface. Determination of the correct orientation of the lenticule in the anterior chamber is essential for surgeons, which is not possible with a routine microscope because the visibility of the anterior chamber remains poor. With the dense corneal edema, this procedure is highly inappropriate in the routine clinical settings. Hence, approaching through the anterior surface of cornea rather than posterior corneal surface is preferable.

18. Conclusion

Management of acute hydrops influences a long-term visual outcome. ASOCT provides a superior insight into the pathogenesis of acute hydrops. An early intervention is essential for preventing the vascularization of the corneal scar and eventually improving the prognosis of penetrating keratoplasty. Compression sutures, intra cameral gas, and a combination of both are efficient techniques described in the literature with a proven efficacy in hastening the resolution of the corneal edema. DALK and mini-DMEK are highly skillful procedures with questionable reproducibility by multiple surgeons. Prevention of acute hydrops should be a primary goal of all corneal surgeons in the future. An early identification and management of progressive keratoconus, prevention of eye rubbing, and avoidance of the professional sports may decrease the incidence of acute hydrops.

Author details

Praveen Subudhi*, Sweta Patro and Nageswar Rao Subudhi
Ruby Eye Hospital, Berhampur, Ganjam, Odisha, India

*Address all correspondence to: subudhipraveen@gmail.com

References

[1] Barsam A, Petrushkin H, Brennan N, et al. Acute corneal hydrops in keratoconus: a national prospective study of incidence and management. Eye (Lond). 2015; 29(4):469-474. doi:10.1038/eye.2014.333

[2] Tuft SJ, Gregory WM, Buckley RJ. Acute corneal hydrops in keratoconus. Ophthalmology. 1994;101(10):1738-1744. doi:10.1016/s0161-6420(94)31110-9

[3] AMSLER M. Bull Soc Belge Ophtalmol. 1961;129:331-354

[4] Fan Gaskin JC, Good WR, Jordan CA, Patel DV, McGhee CNj. The Auckland keratoconus study: identifying predictors of acute corneal hydrops in keratoconus. Clin Exp Optom. 2013;96(2):208-213. doi:10.1111/cxo.12048

[5] Grewal S, Laibson PR, Cohen EJ, Rapuano CJ. Acute hydrops in the corneal ectasias: associated factors and outcomes. Trans Am Ophthalmol Soc. 1999;97:187-203.

[6] Krachmer JH, Feder RS, Belin MW. Keratoconus and related non-inflammatory corneal thinning disorders. SurvOphthalmol. 1984;28: 293-322.

[7] Brunsting LA, Reed WB, Blair HL. Occurrence of cataract and keratoconus with atopic dermatitis. Arch Dermatol 1955;72:237-41

[8] Galin MA, Berger R. Atopy and keratoconus. Am J Ophthalmol 1958;45: 904-6

[9] Spencer WH, Fisher JJ. The association of keratoconus with atopic dermatitis. Am J Ophthalmol 1959;47:332-4.

[10] Bawazeer AM, Hodge WG, Lorimer B. Atopy and keratoconus: A multivariate analysis. Br J Ophthalmol. 2000;84:834-6

[11] Weed KH, MacEwen CJ, Giles T, Low J, McGhee CN. The Dundee University Scottish Keratoconus study: Demographics, corneal signs, associated diseases, and eye rubbing.

[12] Balasubramanian SA, Mohan S, Pye DC, Willcox MD. Proteases, proteolysis and inflammatory molecules in the tears of people with keratoconus. ActaOphthalmol. 2012;90:e303-9.

[13] Balasubramanian SA, Pye DC, Willcox MD. Effects of eye rubbing on the levels of protease, protease activity and cytokines in tears: Relevance in keratoconus. ClinExpOptom. 2013;96:214-8.

[14] Ben-Eli H, Erdinest N, Solomon A. Pathogenesis and complications of chronic eye rubbing in ocular allergy. CurrOpin Allergy ClinImmunol. 2019;19(5):526-534. doi:10.1097/ACI.0000000000000571

[15] Barr JT, Zadnik K, Wilson BS, et al. Factors associated with corneal scarring in the Collaborative Longitudinal Evaluation of Keratoconus (CLEK) Study. Cornea. 2000;19(4):501-507. doi:10.1097/00003226-200007000-00020

[16] di Martino E, Ali M, Inglehearn CF. Matrix metalloproteinases in keratoconus - too much of a good thing? Exp Eye Res 2019; 182:137-143.

[17] Masterton SAM. Mechanobiology of the corneal epithelium. Exp Eye Res 2018; 177:122-129

[18] Korb DR, Finnemor VM, Herman JP. Apical changes and scarring in keratoconus as related to contact lens fitting techniques. J Am OptomAssoc 1982; 53:199-205.

[19] Sharma R, Titiyal JS, Prakash G, Sharma N, Tandon R, Vajpayee RB. Clinical profile and risk factors for keratoplasty and development of hydrops in north Indian patients with keratoconus. Cornea. 2009;28:367-70.

[20] Stoiber J, Muss W, Ruckhofer J, Grabner G. Acute keratoconus with perforation in a patient with Down's syndrome. Br J Ophthalmol. 2003;87:120.

[21] Robertson I. Keratoconus and the Ehlers-Danlos syndrome: a new aspect of keratoconus. Med J Aust. 1975;1(18):571-573.

[22] Tsang SH, Sharma T. Leber Congenital Amaurosis. AdvExp Med Biol. 2018;1085:131-137. doi:10.1007/978-3-319-95046-4_26

[23] Freedman J, Gombos GM. Bilateral macular coloboma, keratoconus, and retinitis pigmentosa. Ann Ophthalmol. 1971;3(6):

[24] Idowu OO, Ashraf DC, Vagefi MR, Kersten RC, Winn BJ. Floppy eyelid syndrome: ocular and systemic associations. Curr Opin Ophthalmol. 2019;30(6):513-524. doi:10.1097/ICU.0000000000000617

[25] Bilgihan K, Hondur A, Sul S, Ozturk S. Pregnancy-induced progression of keratoconus. Cornea. 2011;30(9):991-994. doi:10.1097/ICO.0b013e3182068adc

[26] Fan Gaskin JC, Good WR, Jordan CA, Patel DV, McGhee CNj. The Auckland keratoconus study: identifying predictors of acute corneal hydrops in keratoconus. Clin Exp Optom. 2013;96(2):208-213. doi:10.1111/cxo.12048

[27] Choi JA, Kim MS. Progression of keratoconus by longitudinal assessment with corneal topography. Invest Ophthalmol Vis Sci. 2012;53(2):927-935. Published 2012 Feb 23. doi:10.1167/iovs.11-8118

[28] Shajari M, Steinwender G, Herrmann K, et al. Evaluation of keratoconus progression. Br J Ophthalmol. 2019;103(4):551-557. doi:10.1136/bjophthalmol-2017-311651

[29] Bron AJ. Keratoconus. Cornea. 1988; 7(3):163-169.

[30] Subudhi P, Khan Z, Subudhi BNR, Sitaram S. To show the efficacy of compressive sutures alone in the management of acute hydrops in a keratoconus patient. BMJ Case Rep. 2017;2017:bcr2016218843. Published 2017 May 4. doi:10.1136/bcr-2016-218843

[31] Laing RA, Sandstrom MM, Berrospi AR, Leibowitz HM. The human corneal endothelium in keratoconus: A specular micro-scopic study. Arch Ophthalmol. 1979;97(10):1867-1869. doi:10.1001/archopht.1979.01020020315005

[32] Cameron JA, Al-Rajhi AA, Badr IA. Corneal ectasia in vernal keratoconjunctivitis. Ophthalmology 1989;96(11):1615-1623.

[33] Taboureau E, Berthout A, Turut P, Milazzo S. Dégénérescence marginale pellucide compliquée d'un hydrops cornéenaiguspontané [Acute spontaneous corneal hydrops in a patient with pellucid marginal corneal degeneration]. J Fr Ophtalmol. 2006;29(6):e13. doi:10.1016/s0181-5512(06)73830-x

[34] Rychener RO, Kirby DB. Acute hydrops of the corneal complicating keratoconus. Arch Ophthalmol 1940; 24(2): 326-343.

[35] Tuft SJ, Gregory WM, Buckley RJ. Acute corneal hydrops in keratoconus. Ophthalmology 1994;101(10):1738-1744.

[36] Fan Gaskin JC, Good WR, Jordan CA, Patel DV, McGhee C. The Auckland keratoconus study: identifying predictors of acute corneal hydrops

in keratoconus. ClinExpOptom 2013;96(2):208-213.

[37] Zadnik K, Barr JT, Gordon MO, Edrington TB. Biomicroscopic signs and disease severity in keratoconus. Collaborative Longitudinal Evaluation of Keratoconus (CLEK) Study Group. Cornea 1996; 15: 139-146

[38] Grewal S, Laibson PR, Cohen EJ, Rapuano CJ. Acute hydrops in the corneal ectasias: associated factors and outcomes. Trans Am OphthalmolSoc 1999; 97: 187-198; discussion 198-203.

[39] Rowson NJ, Dart JK, Buckley RJ. Corneal neovascularisation in acute hydrops. Eye 1992;6(4):404-406.

[40] Fuentes E, Sandali O, El Sanharawi M, et al. Anatomic Predictive Factors of Acute Corneal Hydrops in Keratoconus: An Optical Coherence Tomography Study. Ophthalmology. 2015;122(8):1653-1659. doi:10.1016/j.ophtha.2015.04.031

[41] Lockington D, Fan Gaskin JC, McGhee CN, Patel DV. A prospective study of acute corneal hydrops by in vivo confocal microscopy in a New Zealand population with keratoconus. Br J Ophthalmol. 2014;98(9):1296-1302. doi:10.1136/bjophthalmol-2013-304145

[42] Basu, Sayan MS; Vaddavalli, Pravin K. MS; Vemuganti, Geeta K. MD; Hasnat Ali, Md MBA; Murthy, Somasheila I. MS Anterior Segment Optical Coherence Tomography Features of Acute Corneal Hydrops, Cornea: May 2012 - Volume 31 - Issue 5 - p 479-485 doi: 10.1097/ICO.0b013e318223988e

[43] Kallel S, Tahiri Joutei Hassani R, Liang H, Baudouin C, Labbé A. Apport de l'OCT de segment antérieur « en face » dans le kératocôneaigu ["En face" anterior segment optical coherence tomography findings in acute corneal hydrops]. J Fr Ophtalmol. 2014;37(8):605-612

[44] Margo CE, Mosteller MW. Corneal pseudocyst following acute hydrops. Br J Ophthalmol. 1987;71(5):359-360. doi:10.1136/bjo.71.5.359

[45] Sharma N, Mannan R, Jhanji V, et al. Ultrasound biomicroscopy-guided assessment of acute corneal hydrops. Ophthalmology 2011;118(11): 2166-2171. 22.

[46] Feder RS, Wilhelmus KR, Vold SD, O'Grady RB. Intrastromal clefts in keratoconus patients with hydrops. Am J Ophthalmol 1998;126(1):9-16.

[47] Labbé A, Kallel S, Denoyer A, Dupas B, Baudouin C. Imagerie de la cornée[Cornealimaging].JFrOphtalmol. 2012;35(8):628-634. doi:10.1016/j.jfo.2012.02.008

[48] Cruzat A, Qazi Y, Hamrah P. In Vivo Confocal Microscopy of Corneal Nerves in Health and Disease. Ocul Surf. 2017;15(1):15-47. doi:10.1016/j.jtos.2016.09.004

[49] Fuentes E, Sandali O, El Sanharawi M, Basli E, Hamiche T, Goemaere I, Borderie V, Bouheraoua N, Laroche L. Anatomic Predictive Factors of Acute Corneal Hydrops in Keratoconus: An Optical Coherence Tomography Study. Ophthalmology. 2015 Aug;122(8):1653-9. doi: 10.1016/j.ophtha.2015.04.031. Epub 2015 Jun 2. PMID: 26045363.

[50] Rubsamen PE, McLeish WM. Keratoconus with acute hydrops and perforation. Brief case report. Cornea. 1991 Jan;10(1):83-4. PMID: 2019114

[51] .Sharif Z, Sharif W. Corneal neovascularization: updates on pathophysiology, investigations & management. Rom J Ophthalmol. 2019 Jan-Mar;63(1):15-22. PMID: 31198893; PMCID: PMC6531773.

[52] Gonçalves ED, Campos M, Paris F, Gomes JA, Farias CC.

Ceratopatiabolhosa: etiopatogênese e tratamento [Bullous keratopathy: etiopathogenesis and treatment]. Arq Bras Oftalmol. 2008 Nov-Dec;71(6 Suppl):61-4. Portuguese. doi: 10.1590/s0004-27492008000700012. PMID: 19274413

[53] Henry CR, Flynn HW Jr, Miller D, Forster RK, Alfonso EC. Infectious keratitis progressing to endophthalmitis: a 15-year study of microbiology, associated factors, and clinical outcomes. Ophthalmology. 2012 Dec;119(12):2443-9. doi: 10.1016/j.ophtha.2012.06.030. Epub 2012 Aug 1. PMID: 22858123; PMCID: PMC3490005

[54] Connon CJ, Meek KM. The structure and swelling of corneal scar tissue in penetrating full-thickness wounds. Cornea. 2004 Mar;23(2):165-71. doi: 10.1097/00003226-200403000-00010. PMID: 15075886

[55] Pandey N, Chandrakar AK, Garg ML, Patel SS. Calotropisprocera -induced keratitis. Indian J Ophthalmol. 2009 Jan-Feb;57(1):58-60. doi: 10.4103/0301-4738.44492. PMID: 19075415; PMCID: PMC2661522

[56] Arenas E, Mieth A, Muñoz D. Combined intrastromal injection of ganciclovir and depot betamethasone for the management of nummular keratitis: Case series. Arch SocEspOftalmol. 2019 Jul;94(7):347-351. English, Spanish. doi: 10.1016/j.oftal.2019.01.009. Epub 2019 Mar 4. PMID: 30846248

[57] Messmer EM. Keratitis - infektiösoderautoimmun? [Keratitis - Infectious or Autoimmune?]. KlinMonblAugenheilkd. 2016 Jul;233(7):808-12. German. doi: 10.1055/s-0042-105155. Epub 2016 Jul 28. PMID: 27468096

[58] Faith SC, Durrani AF, Jhanji V. Cytomegalovirus keratitis. CurrOpin-Ophthalmol. 2018 Jul;29(4):373-377. doi: 10.1097/ICU.0000000000000481. PMID: 29708927

[59] Zhuang M, Fan W, Xie P, Yuan ST, Liu QH, Zhao C. Evaluation of the safety and quality of day-case cataract surgery based on 4151 cases. Int J Ophthalmol. 2019 Feb 18;12(2):291-295. doi: 10.18240/ijo.2019.02.17. PMID: 30809487; PMCID: PMC6376245

[60] Yuen HK, Rassier CE, Jardeleza MS, Green WR, de la Cruz Z, Stark WJ, Gottsch JD. A morphologic study of Fuchs dystrophy and bullous keratopathy. Cornea. 2005 Apr;24(3):319-27. doi: 10.1097/01.ico.0000148288.53323.b2. PMID: 15778606.

[61] Grewal S, Laibson PR, Cohen EJ, Rapuano CJ. Acute hydrops in the corneal ectasias: associated factors and outcomes. Trans Am OphthalmolSoc 1999;97:187-198

[62] Carter JB, Jones DB, Wilhelmus KR. Acute hydrops in pellucid marginal corneal degeneration. Am J Ophthalmol 1989; 107: 167-170

[63] Panda A, Aggarwal A, Madhavi P, et al. Management of acute corneal hydrops secondary to keratoconus with intracameral injection of sulfur hexafluoride (SF6). Cornea 2007;26(9):1067-1069.

[64] Basu S, Vaddavalli PK, Ramappa M, Shah S, Murthy SI, Sangwan VS. Intracameral perfluoropropane gas in the treatment of acute corneal hydrops. Ophthalmology 2011;118(5):934-939.

[65] Li S, Liu M, Wang Q, Wang T, Shi W. Lamellar keratoplasty following thermokeratoplasty in the treatment of acute corneal hydrops. Am J Ophthalmol. 2014 Jul;158(1):26-31.e1. doi: 10.1016/j.ajo.2014.03.011. Epub 2014 Mar 31. PMID: 24699158.

[66] Jacob S, Narasimhan S, Agarwal A, Sambath J, Umamaheshwari G,

Saijimol AI. Primary Modified Predescemetic Deep Anterior Lamellar Keratoplasty in Acute Corneal Hydrops. Cornea. 2018 Oct;37(10):1328-1333. doi: 10.1097/ICO.0000000000001693. PMID: 30001263.

[67] Bachmann B, Händel A, Siebelmann S, Matthaei M, Cursiefen C. Mini-Descemet Membrane Endothelial Keratoplasty for the Early Treatment of Acute Corneal Hydrops in Keratoconus. Cornea. 2019 Aug;38(8):1043-1048. doi: 10.1097/ICO.0000000000002001. PMID: 31276462

Chapter 2

Femto Laser-Assisted Cataract Surgery

Clemence Bonnet, Saba Al-Hashimi, Antoine P. Brézin and Dominique Monnet

Abstract

Cataract is a leading cause of blindness in the world, and cataract extraction is one of the most commonly performed surgeries. Preferred surgical techniques have changed over the past decades with associated improvements in outcomes and safety. Phacoemulsification is a highly successful technique first introduced over 40 years ago. It is the current method of cataract surgery, with a very low reported rate of major complications and a frequency of overall intraoperative complications of less than 2%. Application of the femtosecond laser evolved to now assist in cataract surgery and has been termed FLACS (femtosecond laser-assisted cataract surgery) and occurs in three steps: corneal incisions (including optional limbal relaxing incisions to reduce astigmatism), anterior capsulotomy, and lens fragmentation. The remaining surgical steps still require the surgeon's hands. The FLACS technique may have some advantages compared with conventional phacoemulsification. It remains however unclear whether FLACS is globally more efficient and safer than conventional surgery. The popularity of FLACS may also be limited by its higher cost compared with conventional surgery. The potential advantages of laser-assisted surgery are yet to be determined as FLACS technology is relatively new and in continuous evolution. This chapter reports scientific data as well as our own experience with this new technology. All the platforms currently available are described.

Keywords: cataract surgery, femtosecond laser, phacoemulsification, FLACS (femtosecond laser-assisted cataract surgery)

1. Introduction

Techniques in cataract surgery have been dramatically progressing over the past half-century with associated improvements in outcomes and safety [1, 2]. Manual phacoemulsification remains the most popular technique in developed countries, representing about 90% of procedures [3]. Although a number of recent developments have occurred in intraocular lens technology, the basic phacoemulsification procedure has remained unchanged over the past 20 years [4, 5].

"Femto" is a prefix of the International System of Units that stands for 10^{-15}, a millionth of a billionth. The femtosecond laser consists of a solid-state laser source that emits impulses of a wavelength close to the infrared spectrum with a duration measurement in femtoseconds. Its emission frequency is 10,000 pulses per second of monochromatic light. Corneal flap creation during laser in situ keratomileusis (LASIK) is the most common use of this laser [6, 7]. The latest innovation is its use in cataract surgery, called FLACS (femto laser-assisted cataract surgery) [8, 9]. The recent introduction of femtosecond laser to cataract surgery, by Nagy et al. in 2008, and its Food and Drug Administration (FDA) approval in 2010 represents a potentially significant advancement in cataract technology, with expectations of greater safety and better visual outcomes [10–12].

2. Femtosecond laser principles

The femtosecond laser has a similar action to the *Nd:YAG* laser used in pseudophakic capsulotomies. The Nd:YAG laser and the femtosecond laser have nearly identical wavelengths, respectively 1.064 and 1.053 nm. The femtosecond laser light pulses are shorter than the impulse of the Nd: YAG laser, which is on the order of nanoseconds (**Table 1**).

Photodisruption starts with a process called laser induced optical break-down (LIOB), which occurs when conditions of high frequency laser pulses are highly focused with short duration and applied through a small beam laser diameter [13]. The LIOB generates a high-intensity electrical field. The laser pulses cause ionization, meaning the breaking of the bonds between electrons and atomic nuclei, which is responsible for a cavitation bubble phenomenon, related to the expansion of this plasma consisting of ions [14]. This plasma complex will tend to expand at supersonic speed, separating tissue in its path, rapidly losing energy and vaporizing tiny quantities of corneal tissue. The cavitation bubble consists of CO_2, N_2 and H_2O molecules, which are absorbed by the corneal pump mechanism or eliminated when the corneal flap is raised or the eye opened [15]. These ultrafast pulses are too brief to transfer heat and generate inflammation to the tissue, and therefore are considered particularly adapted to cleave tissue. Hundreds of thousands of adjacent pulses can shape uniform horizontal, vertical or oblique cut surfaces. The pulses are always emitted from the deepest targeted layers of the cornea toward the most superficial ones, to avoid the generated cavitation bubbles from stopping laser pulses focused on the underlying layers. One of fundamental requirement for femtolaser intervention is corneal transparency, allowing precise focus of the laser spots and energy delivery.

The femtosecond laser used in cataract surgery has been specifically developed for the following surgical steps: main and accessory corneal incisions, capsulorhexis, lens fragmentation, and optional arcuate incisions for intraoperative correction of astigmatism. The depth of treatment can reach 8 mm, from the corneal epithelium to lens posterior capsule. The pulsed energy used by a femtosecond laser for cataract surgery is on a scale of microjoules (μJ) and 15 μJ is the maximum energy of pulses.

Laser	Wavelength (nm)	Effect on tissue
Carbon dioxide	10600, far infrared	Photothermal
Nd:YAG	1064, near infrared	Photodisruption
Femtosecond	1053, near infrared	Photodisruption
Krypton	647-531, visible light	Photochemical coagulation
Argon	614-488, visible light	Photochemical coagulation
Excimer	193, far ultraviolet	Photoablation

Table 1.
Use of lasers in ophthalmology.

3. Platforms available and procedure

Five FLACS devices are currently available:

- LenSx (Alcon LenSx, Inc., Aliso Viejo, CA, USA)
- LensAR (LENSAR, Inc., Winter Park, FL, USA)
- Catalys (OptiMedica, Abbott Medical Optics, Santa Clara, CA, USA)
- Victus (Technolas Perfect Vision and Bausch and Lomb, Rochester, NY, USA)
- LDV Z8 (Ziemer Ophthalmic Systems AG, Port, Switzerland)

The laser programming consists in individual steps: (1) customize the treatment with the graphic user interface, (2) dock with patient interface, (3) image via OCT scan, (4) analyze the image and (5) treat with the femtosecond laser. These functions are clustered on a computer supplied with the femtosecond laser (and the patient bed, depending on the device). The association of the femtosecond laser, the graphic user interface, the docking system, and the OCT scan constitutes the femtolaser platform. Femtolaser platforms are quite similar to each other and are fitted either with an optical coherence tomography (OCT) imaging system or a Scheimpflug camera to guide the laser beam to the target. Recording of patient data and customized profiles are made through the touchscreen monitor. Platforms differ in step order, docking interface, lens fragmentation patterns and speed of action (**Table 2**). The environmental needs for the laser system are crucial to provide reproducible procedures. The space in the operative room must be considered as the devices occupies between 2 and 3 m^3 (except the LDV Z8, which is a smaller portable device) and must be near to the phacoemulsifier. **Table 3** summarizes these requirements.

	LenSx	**LensAR**	**Catalys**	**Victus**	**LDV Z8**
	Alcon	**LensAR**	**AMO**	**Bausch & Lomb, Technolas**	**Ziemer**
Room size (m)	3.4 × 4.3	4.57 × 4.57	3.04 × 3.35	3.4 × 3.7	No specific needs
Laser size (h × l × p, m)	Screen: 1.22 × 0.76 × 0.61; laser: 0.51 × 0.58 × 0.20	1.65 × 1.97 × 0.8	1.15 × 1.64 × 0.84	1.67 × 2.1 × 0.82	1.4 × 1 × 0.6
Docking	Curved applanation lens	Fluid-fill suction ring	Fluid-fill suction ring	Curved applanation lens	Fluid-fill suction ring + curved applanation lens
Imaging	HD-OCT	HD-OCT + Scheimpflug camera	HD-OCT	HD-OCT	HD-OCT
Included bed	No	No	Yes	Yes	No
Corneal refractive procedure	Yes	No	No	Yes	Yes

Table 2.
FLACS platforms available.

Docking the eye to the system means connecting the eye to the laser. This is done via a patient interface. The patient interface utilizes suction to stabilize the eye and maintain a clear optical pathway for imaging and laser delivery. The goal during suction is to obtain a clear and stable image during the laser treatment while controlling the increased intra ocular pressure and the image quality. Each platform has a specific patient interface, for example, with the Catalys, docking is accomplished with a liquid filled interface which allowed a good cornea visualization during docking. The LenSx uses a curved applanated interface, which can create posterior corneal folds which can interfere with the ability to image and cut tissue effectively. Optimal docking is achieved when there is a symmetric scleral show.

3.1 LenSX

The LenSX laser is a standard unit that does not require external connections to water or gas. Recent updates have changed the diameter of the patient-interface, now called SoftFit PI, which allowed a 20% reduction in intraocular pressure (IOP), providing less discomfort for the patient (**Figure 1**). The SoftFit® interface has a soft lens insert in the interface that allows the reduction of corneal folds during the docking, and a better delivery of the laser beam [16]. The integrated anterior segment optical coherence tomography OCT provides real-time scanning from the corneal epithelium to the posterior lens capsule with a high-resolution video. This imaging system is able to either take a single OCT snapshot, or produce live continuous OCT images (**Figures 2–4**). Thanks to live OCT, surgeons can immediately check if the patient's positioning is adequate, reducing the risk of tilt during the docking procedure.

3.2 LensAR

The LENSAR docking system is a noncontact disposable fluid filled patient. The suction ring is low pressure, which decreases the frequency of subconjunctival

Operating temperature of the environment	18–24°C
Operating humidity	30–65%
24-hour air conditioning system sterility	
Class A operating room (minor surgery under topical or local anesthesia)	
Handwashing facilities	
Smooth and washable floors	

Table 3.
Environmental requirements for the laser system set-up space.

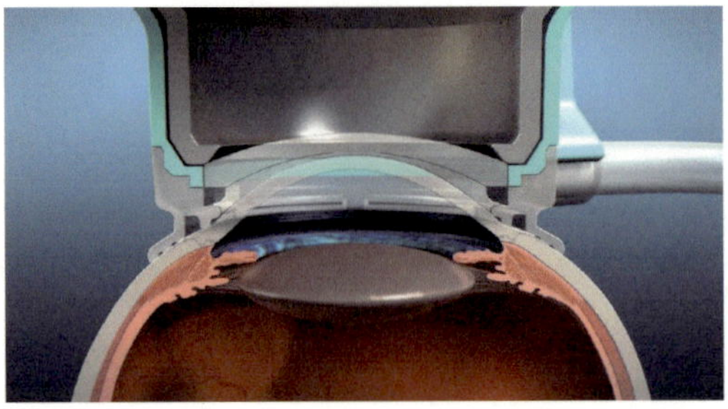

Figure 1.
LensX docking system, SofFit® interface.

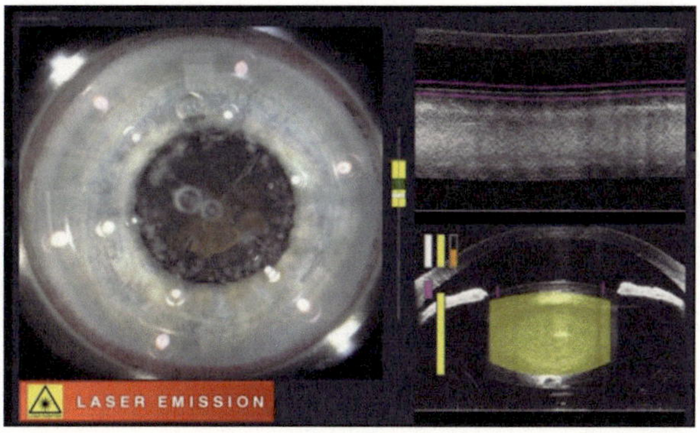

Figure 2.
LensX capsulotomy procedure.

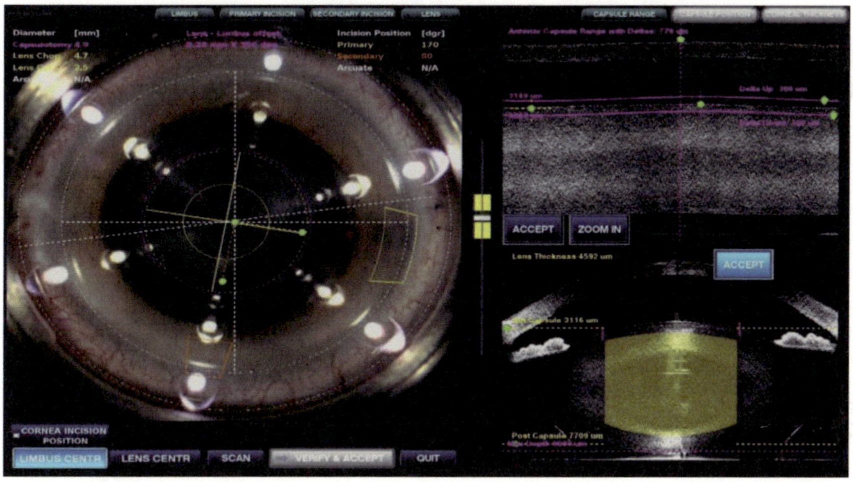

Figure 3.
LensX incisions procedure.

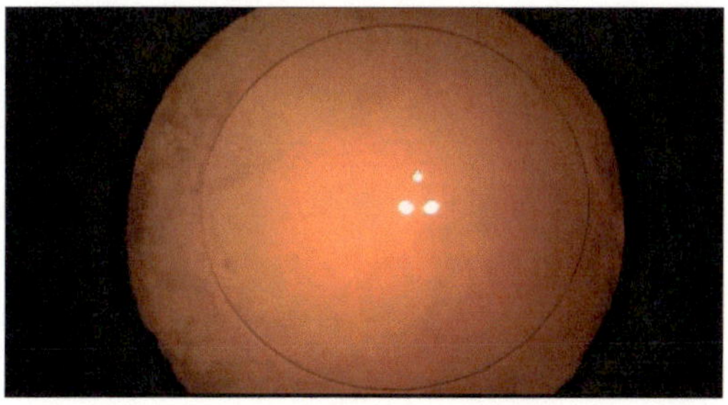

Figure 4.
Free floating continuous, curvilinear, and circular capsulotomy with LensX.

hemorrhages and minimizes the risk of high intraocular pressure. The system includes a Scheimpflug three-dimensional confocal system combined with a laser biometric system allowing scans of the anterior segment at varying speeds. The depth-of-field imaging is enhanced compared with OCT technology. The nuclear fragmentation consists of radial sections or concentric cylindrical cuts and allows cubic, spherical or pie-cut patterns. The system is also able to detect and compensate for tilt (**Figure 5**).

3.3 Catalys

The docking system, called "Liquid Optics®," includes two parts: one is fitted to the patient by suction and the second couples to the first cone to the console of the Catalys optics system. The suction ring, which is filled with a balanced saline solution (BSS), requires a vacuum that does not exceed 15 mm Hg. The OCT images are guided through a continuous optical system. The system software identifies the ocular surfaces, reconstructs areas to be excluded from laser treatment and customizes the treatment according to the observed structures.

The patterns of lens fragmentation are wide and allow control of grid spacing (from 100 to 2000 μm) (**Figures 6–9**).

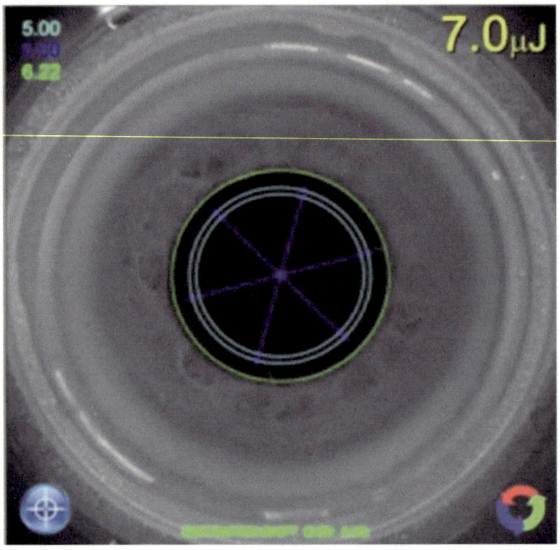

Figure 5.
LensAR lens fragmentation patterns.

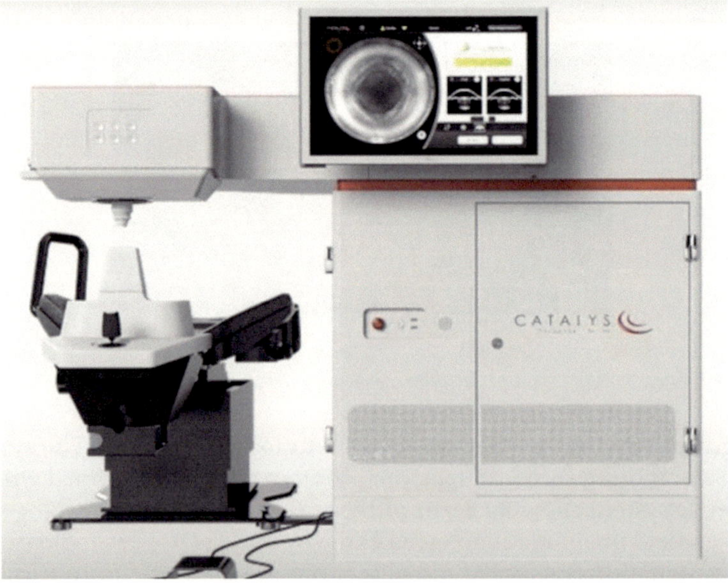

Figure 6.
Catalys device.

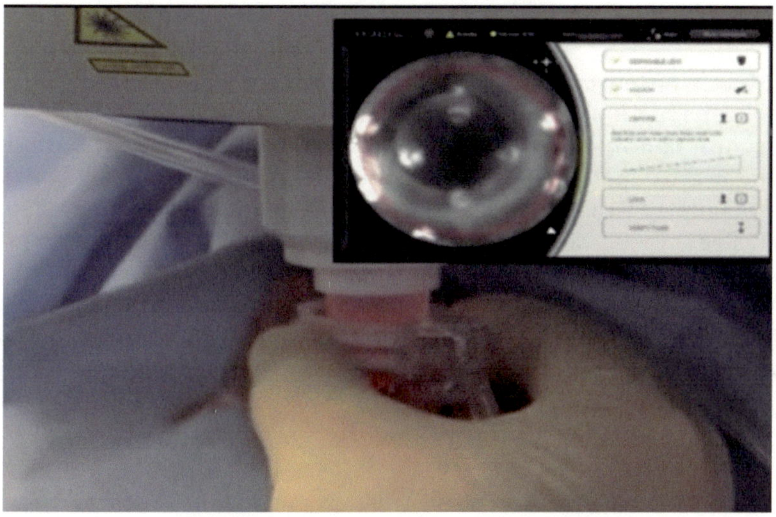

Figure 7.
Liquid optics® Interface.

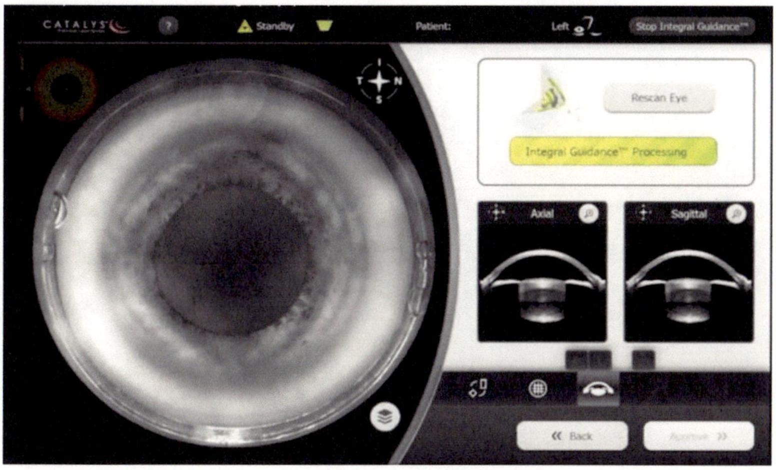

Figure 8.
Per-operative CATALYS visualization.

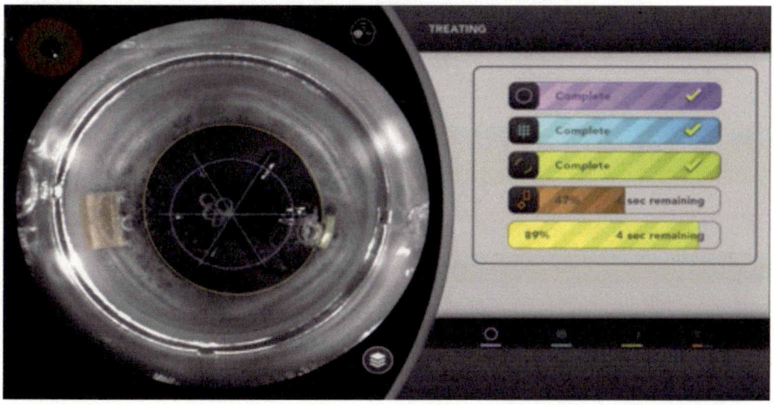

Figure 9.
Laser treatment with CATALYS.

3.4 VICTUS

The VICTUS system currently uses two components for laser docking: a low-pressure silicone suction ring and a curved interface cone. Adaptation of the curved interface cone is controlled by intelligent sensors, which change pressure levels exerted on the eye depending on the treatment. The image capturing system is a spectral-domain OCT that takes real-time images and identifies anterior segment structures. The surgeon can manually locate the area of photodisruption in the nucleus and its distance to the posterior capsule.

Flaps in refractive corneal procedures and incisions are also possible, making it a versatile femtosecond laser system. The laser source operates at 80 kHz for the FLACS procedure. The optical-acoustic-modulator included allows modulation in the laser pulses' frequency: it can change from 80 kHz for the FLACS procedure to 160 kHz for the LASIK-flap procedure (**Figures 10–12**).

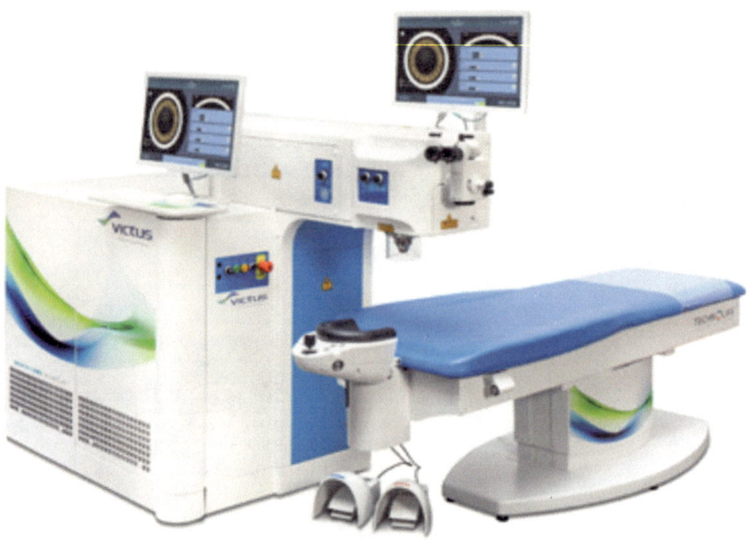

Figure 10.
VICTUS device.

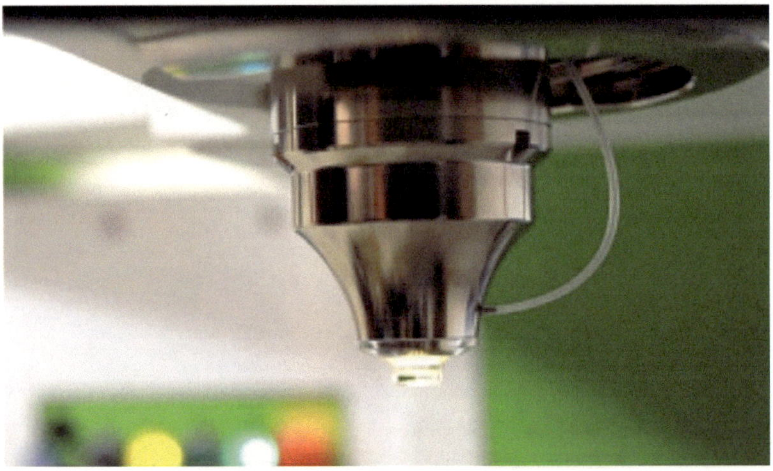

Figure 11.
VICTUS docking system.

3.5 LDV Z8

The device is the first mobile cataract femtosecond laser that can be easily suit in the operating room. Ziemer has developed a liquid-filled nonapplanating interface which adheres to the eye with minimal suction and thus avoids corneal folds. The FEMTO LDV Z8 employs a combination of two imaging systems for real-time visual control of the docking process and of the positioning of dissections: the TopView®, a high-definition camera which provides visual control of the alignment of the patient

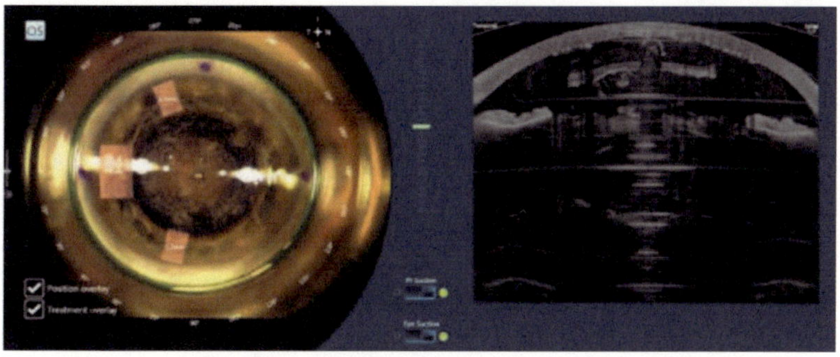

Figure 12.
VICTUS laser treatment with free floating capsulotomy.

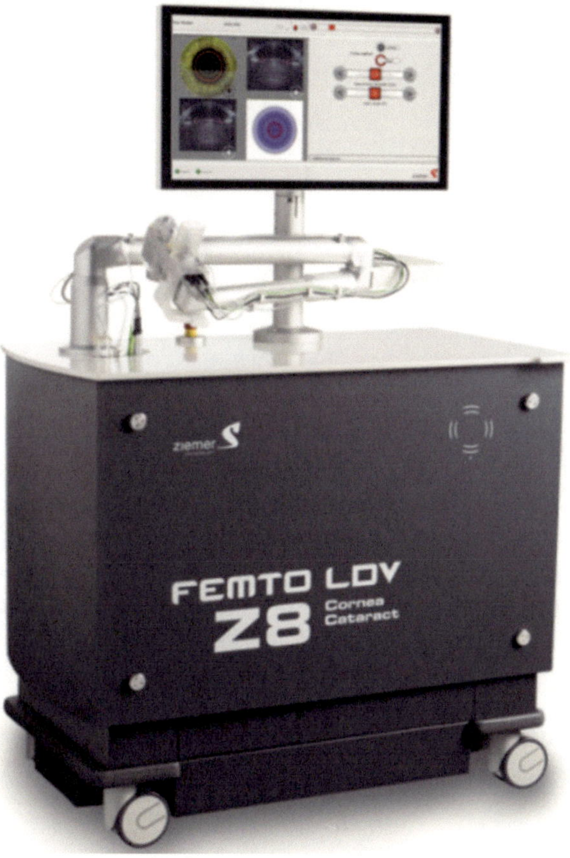

Figure 13.
LDV Z8 device.

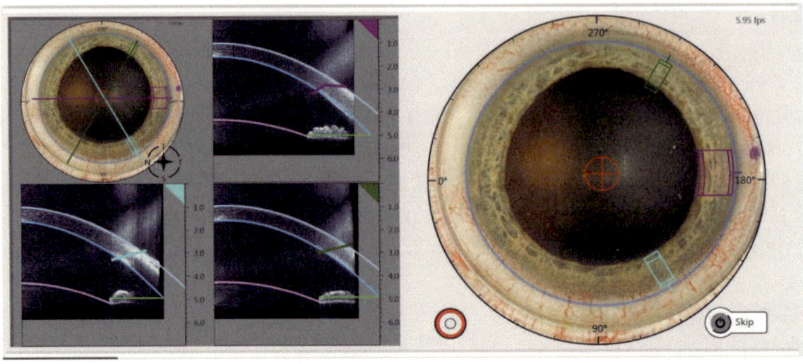

Figure 14.
LDV Z8 procedure and incisions.

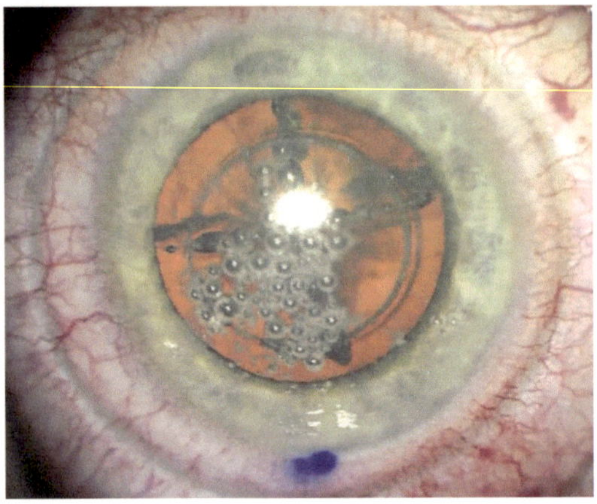

Figure 15.
Eye after LDV Z8 procedure.

interface to the eye and a proprietary OCT system, operating in the near-infrared range (**Figures 13–15**) [17]. It obtained FDA approval for FLACS in 2016.

3.6 Procedure

Proper docking requires cooperation from the patient. The liquid interface has advantages of causing less tissue distortion and minimal increase in intraocular pressure as well as less mean eye movement during capsulotomy. The cornea should be well centered in the patient interface before docking to avoid misalignment of corneal incisions. Apart from the transient learning curve, docking may cause subconjunctival hemorrhage [18]. The estimated incidence of this side effect is 34% and significantly decreased using the liquid interface device with lower suction pressure, and shorter treatment time [19].

4. Description of the intervention

4.1 Capsulotomy

The capsulotomy cut opens the lens's anterior capsule in a continuous, curvilinear, and circular fashion with high precision to improve safety during intraocular maneuvers. We advise to choose a 5.2 mm diameter capsulotomy, with a delta up at

400 μm and a delta down of 350 μm. The energy recommended is 15 μJ, with a 4 μm spot separation and a 3 μm layer separation. Laser capsulotomies have been shown to be better centered than manual continuous curvilinear capsulorhexis (CCC), with highly predictable sizes [20–22].

4.1.1 Lens fragmentation

The surgeon defines the pattern, the length, and the number of cuts. The energy level, the anterior and posterior lens capsule parameters, pattern separation and the primary incision angle have to be specified. Then, the nucleus can be easily split.

4.1.2 Limbal relaxing incisions

It is possible to correct a small amount of astigmatism (<1.5 D) with arcuate incisions (AI) [23]. Nomograms can facilitate surgical planning by determining the proper treatment for an intended correction [24]. Arcuate incisions can be left unopened until the postoperative period depending on the postoperative refractive error [25].

4.1.3 Corneal incision

All corneal incisions are placed just inside the limbus. The real-time anterior segment imaging provides the peripheral corneal thickness at the location of the incision during the procedure. We recommend a 2.2 mm three planes (90°/11°/90°) main incision at 135° and a one plane 1.2 mm incision at 5° for the side-port incision. The spot the layer separation should be 4 μm with an energy level of 5.5 μJ.

4.2 After the laser procedure

After removing the docking system, next steps are similar to manual phacoemulsification. The cortex aspiration can be tricky because the femtosecond laser cut it just below the capsulotomy. If the irrigation/aspiration probe is not sufficient, a Simcoe cannula can be used. To help, the cortex may be washed with a 25G syringe full of balanced salt solution.

4.3 Complications

4.3.1 Suction break

Sudden suction break can occur in less than 2% of cases, but did not lead to further complications as laser treatment can be started over (**Table 4**) [19]. Most important factors to prevent it are precise patient interface placement and good preoperative anesthesia. Hard headrest avoids the head from being pushed down during insertion of the patient interface and reduces the risk for suction loss.

4.3.2 Pupillary constriction

The incidence of pupillary constriction is 19% and arises during the first steps of the femtolaser procedure [19]. The laser application itself can cause pupillary miosis. Bubble formation in the anterior chamber releases small amounts of free radicals and prostaglandins that can trigger pupillary constriction. Highly myopic eyes and eyes with pseudoexfoliation syndrome are prone to a miotic reaction after femtosecond laser treatment. Intracameral epinephrine before lens removal can help enlarge the pupil and facilitate the surgery [26]. Iris hooks, retractors or a

Conjunctival hemorrhage	34%
Pupillary constriction	19%
Suction break	2%
Capsule complications	2%
Posterior rupture	0.53–1.9%
Anterior tear	0.02%
Block syndrome	0.001%
Endothelial damages	0.002%
Wrong corneal incison localization	0.002%

Table 4.
Rate of complications.

Malyugin ring can be placed after the laser procedure if miosis results. In a case of insufficient mydriasis and an ectopic pupil, Malyugin et al. have developed a surgical technique that combines use of an iris hook and a pupil expansion ring followed by FLACS [27]. Prophylaxis may be an adapted management of the procedure. If the patient is operated immediately after the femtolaser, the prostaglandins released hardly have the time to have effect on the sphincter pupillae. Moreover, pupil dilatation should start 1 hour before, with more frequent instillation of mydriatics.

4.3.3 Capsule complications

4.3.3.1 Incomplete capsulorhexis and anterior capsule tear

A recent meta-analysis shows that the number of anterior capsule and posterior capsule tears for both FLACS and manual phacoemulsification cataract surgery are low, around 0.02% [2]. Tilt, improper docking, loss of suction, corneal folds, and imaging or programming errors can cause partial a capsulotomy. Capsule tags and bridges are usually harmless if they are detected early [28]. The crucial step for capsulotomy removal is to follow the line of the femtosecond laser cut. The absence of a gutter and the presence of bubbles trapped under the capsulotomy cut are signs that help the surgeon identify minor remaining capsule attachments. The surgeon should never pull toward the center of the micro adhesion area because it can cause tags which may run out toward the periphery during hydrodissection or phacoemulsification. One should detach it capsule circumferentially following the contour of the capsulotomy. As small tags can be difficult to see, pulling out the entire anterior capsule with sudden movement is not recommended.

When an anterior capsule tear occurs, the surgeon should perform a very gentle hydrodissection and the canula should be placed 90 degrees from the tear. Avoiding the area of the anterior capsule tear and nucleus rotation is highly advised. During IOL implantation, the leading haptic should be kept away from the tear line.

4.3.3.2 Capsular block syndrome

Capsular block syndrome (CBS) is a rare (0.001%) but serious complication [19]. If hydrodissection with a high-speed influx of fluid is performed, the gas contained in the nucleus cannot access to the anterior chamber, creating an acute intra-capsular high pressure. The subsequent capsular high pressure may lead to a posterior capsular rupture with dropped nucleus. The main signs are the quick constriction of the iris, iris prolapse through the main incision, wrinkling of the capsule and tilting of the lens. Surgeons should be aware of this complication and avoid it by releasing the gas and decompressing the capsular bag before starting hydrodissection. The nucleus may be gently rocked to allow this gas to be burped out. This rock'n roll technique allows air bubbles to leave the crystalline lens. When the gas bubbles leave the intralenticular plane toward the anterior chamber or leave the eye completely, there is no further danger of CBS or posterior capsular rupture.

4.3.3.3 Posterior capsular rupture

Half of posterior capsular tears and lens dislocations are caused by posterior extension of an anterior radial tear. It is imperative that the notches at the anterior capsular margin are recognized and managed during the capsulotomy removal. Completing nuclear fracture centrally to allow any retrolenticular gas to escape is advised. In case of posterior capsular rupture, the management should be the same as during a manual phacoemulsification.

In the first studies, the capsular complication rate during the learning curve (first 200 FLACS procedures) was 7.5% and then decreased to 0.62% (consecutive 1300 cases) [29, 30]. The overall incidence of posterior capsular tears was 3.5% and that of posterior lens dislocation was 2% [30]. In more recent studies, posterior capsular tears have been reported to vary between 0.53 and 1.9%, whereas the incidence of a dropped nucleus has been reported to be between 0.1 and 0.12% [31]. The debate is ongoing: in a recent meta-analysis, Day et al., including 1700 eyes, found that FLACS did not significantly lower the rate of posterior capsular rupture, which was very low in both the FLACS group and manual phacoemulsification group [2]. Though, Popovic et al., including 15,000 eyes, showed that FLACS was associated with higher rates of posterior capsular tears (risk ratio 3.73, $p < 0.05$) [32]. In both studies, the incidence was very low (0.02%) [32]. FLACS might be safer than manual phacoemulsification: lately, Scott et al published the first study with a statistically significant decrease of vitreous loss rate in the FLACS group compared with manual phacoemulsification group (0.65 vs. 1.65%) with a decrease in the individual surgeon's vitreous loss rate [29].

4.3.4 Endothelial damage

Endothelial damage during capsulotomy should be considered as a serious complication of femtosecond laser treatment. This complication was likely caused by the lack of an integrated OCT system with the first devices. Highly hyperopic eyes with a shallow anterior chamber require closer attention to avoid endothelial cuts. In the published cases, the overall incidence was very low (0.002%) and there were no long-term visual consequences of this complication although the endothelial incision line could be observed 1 year after surgery [19].

4.3.5 Wrong corneal incision localization

During corneal wound creation with the femtosecond laser system, if the wound is too central, it can cause surgically induced astigmatism. On the opposite, if the wound is too peripheral, it cannot be opened. Since real-time OCT devices allow visual control of the procedure, the incidence of this complication has dramatically decreased to become very rare (0.002%) [32].

4.4 Personal experience and tips for success

In our experience, with the new platforms, all capsulotomies are complete and we have not seen capsular tears. Depending of the device, the docking is relatively easy. The Catalys device, with its Liquid Optic Interface allows for easy docking without posterior corneal folds. Laser induced miosis can be managed by adding 0.5% tropicamide drops in the liquid filled into the patient interface. We have not seen capsular blockage syndrome as we gently rock the nucleus to remove the gas bubbles trapped into the capsule before performing hydrodissection. We recommend the hydrodissection to be soft but complete. Phacoemulsification is easier after laser treatment but should be performed cautiously by the beginner. All the fragment patterns among the different devices effectively cut the nucleus and allow for easy disassembly. The ice-cube pattern available with the Victus is for us the more efficient pattern, as the surgeon only has to separate the first ice cubes to quickly remove all the nucleus.

TIPS FOR SUCCESS

- Verify the eye's centration (avoid tilting)
- Verify complete capsulotomy
- Evacuate the air bubble before hydrodissection
- Gentle hydrodissection and slow nucleus rotation
- Lens removal: Phaco-chop more than Divide and Conquer
- Cortex removal: Easier if the posterior lens off-set is small (800 μm)

In conclusion, FLACS increases the ease and predictability of the steps involved in cataract surgery but has a surgical learning curve and most of the complications occur during the first 100 procedures [19]. Greater surgeon experience and improved technology are associated with a significant reduction in complications. Most complications are predictable and largely preventable.

5. Safety and efficacy of FLACS

5.1 Intraocular energy delivered

By using a laser to fragment the crystalline lens, less US energy is required to complete its removal. The reduction in the effective phako time can reach 70% and zero phacoemulsification time is possible in nearly 50% of operations [13].

Lower endothelial cell loss with the laser-assisted procedure compared with the manual phacoemulsification has been reported in the early post-operative state due to the reduction of EPT, with the LensX, the LensAR, the Catalys, and the Victus platforms [33].

5.2 Refractive outcomes

5.2.1 Distance visual acuity

The clinical comparative studies performed on a selected series of cases have failed to demonstrate any statistical significance of FLACS versus conventional phacoemulsification surgery concerning the visual outcomes, the intraocular lens power predictability, the corrected distance visual acuity (CDVA) and the uncorrected distance visual acuity (UDVA). Some studies reported better CDVA, UDVA and intraocular lens power predictability for FLACS, while others have reported no differences. In all cases, the 12-month post-operative visual acuity is high. The mean CDVA was 0.03 logMAR, range of −0.08 to 0.05 logMAR [2, 13, 32]. Superiority of UDVA in has been reported at 2 hours, 3 days, and 1 week postoperatively. After 1 month and later, no statistically significant differences between groups are shown [16]. The mean long-term UDVA was 0.13 logMAR, range 0.07 to 0.23 [32, 34].

5.3 Post-operative and long-term complications

5.3.1 Anterior segment inflammation and flare

Two studies demonstrated that postoperative aqueous flare was significantly greater in eyes that had undergone manual cataract surgery at 1 day and at 4 weeks postoperatively than in eyes after FLACS [35, 36] without significant differences regarding retinal thickness after 3 months.

5.3.2 Late capsulorhexis decentration

Compared with manual capsulorhexis, there is evidence of advantages with FLACS by obtaining a more precise shape and size of capsulotomy [22]. This should be associated with a better intraocular lens centration, and then potentially less intraocular lens tilt. However, femtosecond laser capsulotomy shape changes over time and does not improve visual acuity compared with the manual procedure [37].

5.3.3 Vitreoretinal complications

Clinical cystoid macular edema (CME) after cataract surgery, manual or FLACS, remains a rare complication with a prevalence lower than 2% [2]. The peri-operative use of nonsteroidal drops may interfere with the CME rate. Endophthalmitis, expulsive hemorrhage and retinal detachment are rarer complications, estimated at less than 0.1% [38]. No difference between manual phacoemulsification and femtosecond procedures has been described.

5.3.4 Elevated intraocular pressure

The FLACS procedure induces a transient increase of intra-ocular pressure (IOP), during the suction phase, higher with flat and curved applanating contact interfaces compared with the fluid-filled interface. In the 2 years follow-up, no significant elevated IOP was observed after FLACS [39].

In summary, the rate of intra-operative and post-operative complications remains low, less than 2% and not statistically different between FLACS and manual phacoemulsification [40]. Although anterior and posterior capsule tears could have been a concern, the safety of FLACS and phacoemulsification cataract surgery seems equal, considering all complications.

5.4 Cost and resource use

Costs related to FLACS have been much higher than with the conventional procedure so far. It can represent a barrier to wider acceptance by surgeons and clinical centers. This may be difficulty to adopt as more functional benefits have not been yet clearly established with this new technology. An extra-cost of approximately USD 500 to USD 600 per operated eye is associated with FLACS (approximately USD 400,000 for the device, plus USD 150 to 300 for disposables per procedure). However, these elements may vary dramatically among different countries. If FLACS becomes more common in cataract surgery, these costs should decrease. Moreover, sharing a femtolaser platform between several surgeons and/or for several refractive procedures are also a current option to reduce costs [41].

5.5 Advantages and disadvantages of FLACS

Advantages of FLACS over manual phacoemulsification are its precision and predictability regarding the capsulotomy size and centration, corneal wound construction, and nucleus fragmentation [42]. It may be helpful in difficult situations such as pediatric cataracts white or subluxated cataracts. Even if the total energy delivered in the anterior chamber appears lower than during manual phacoemulsification, there is no strong evidence of difference in term of endothelial cell loss between the procedures. The FLACS procedure requires more operating room space as well as increase in operating time. The treatment can also lead to miosis. Altogether, there is no evidence of superior post-operative visual acuity with FLACS, whereas the costs associated with FLACS platforms are currently higher than with manual surgery. Future research on outcomes will help clarify if the increased costs can be supported by evidence of visual and clinical superiority of FLACS.

6. Conclusion: what is the future for FLACS?

The femtosecond laser cataract can be considered a young technology still in significant progress, compared with phacoemulsification, a very mature procedure, which has evolved for decades and has reached a very high level. Each year, companies offer new software evolving to a more user-friendly interface and more efficient versions. Progress is expected in the miniaturization of lasers, making them more moveable. New lenses may be specially designed, based on its perfect laser rhexis and would open a new refractive era, giving significant advantages to the laser procedure. The cost effectiveness is still questioned; many countries cannot afford or consider adopting this technology yet. If adequate improvements are achieved in the "FLACS of the future," this technique may become the gold standard one day.

Conflict of interest

The authors have no financial interests.

Author details

Clemence Bonnet[1,2], Saba Al-Hashimi[2], Antoine P. Brézin[1] and Dominique Monnet[1*]

1 OphtalmoPôle, Hôpital Cochin, APHP, Université de Paris, France

2 Stein Eye Institute, David Geffen School of Medicine, University of Los Angeles, Los Angeles, United States

*Address all correspondence to: dominique.monnet@aphp.fr

References

[1] Clark A, Morlet N, Ng JQ, Preen DB, Semmens JB. Whole population trends in complications of cataract surgery over 22 years in Western Australia. Ophthalmology. 2011;**118**(6):1055-1061

[2] Day AC, Gore DM, Bunce C, Evans JR. Laser-assisted cataract surgery versus standard ultrasound phacoemulsification cataract surgery. Cochrane Database of Systematic Reviews. 2016;7:CD010735

[3] de Silva SR, Riaz Y, Evans JR. Phacoemulsification with posterior chamber intraocular lens versus extracapsular cataract extraction (ECCE) with posterior chamber intraocular lens for age-related cataract. Cochrane Database of Systematic Reviews. 2014;**1**:CD008812

[4] Kessel L, Andresen J, Erngaard D, Flesner P, Tendal B, Hjortdal J. Indication for cataract surgery. Do we have evidence of who will benefit from surgery? A systematic review and meta-analysis. Acta Ophthalmologica. 2016;**94**(1):10-20

[5] Erie JC, Baratz KH, Hodge DO, Schleck CD, Burke JP. Incidence of cataract surgery from 1980 through 2004: 25-year population-based study. Journal of Cataract and Refractive Surgery. 2007;**33**(7):1273-1277

[6] Chen S, Feng Y, Stojanovic A, Jankov MR, Wang Q. IntraLase femtosecond laser vs mechanical microkeratomes in LASIK for myopia: A systematic review and meta-analysis. Journal of Refractive Surgery (Thorofare, N.J.: 1995). 2012;**28**(1):15-24

[7] Torky MA, Al Zafiri YA, Khattab AM, Farag RK, Awad EA. Visumax femtolasik versus Moria M2 microkeratome in mild to moderate myopia: Efficacy, safety, predictability, aberrometric changes and flap thickness predictability. BMC Ophthalmology. 2017;**17**(1):125

[8] Sugar A. Ultrafast (femtosecond) laser refractive surgery. Current Opinion in Ophthalmology. 2002;**13**(4):246-249

[9] He L, Sheehy K, Culbertson W. Femtosecond laser-assisted cataract surgery. Current Opinion in Ophthalmology. 2011;**22**(1):43-52

[10] Nagy Z, Takacs A, Filkorn T, Sarayba M. Initial clinical evaluation of an intraocular femtosecond laser in cataract surgery. Journal of Refractive Surgery (Thorofare, N.J.: 1995). 2009;**25**(12):1053-1060

[11] Aristeidou A, Taniguchi EV, Tsatsos M, Muller R, McAlinden C, Pineda R, et al. The evolution of corneal and refractive surgery with the femtosecond laser. Eye and Vision (London, England). 2015;**2**:12

[12] Ahn H, Kim J-K, Kim CK, Han GH, Seo KY, Kim EK, et al. Comparison of laser in situ keratomileusis flaps created by 3 femtosecond lasers and a microkeratome. Journal of Cataract and Refractive Surgery. 2011;**37**(2):349-357

[13] Grewal DS, Schultz T, Basti S, Dick HB. Femtosecond laser-assisted cataract surgery--Current status and future directions. Survey of Ophthalmology. 2016;**61**(2):103-131

[14] Alió JL, Abdou AA, Soria F, Javaloy J, Fernández-Buenaga R, Nagy ZZ, et al. Femtosecond laser cataract incision morphology and corneal higher-order aberration analysis. Journal of Refractive Surgery (Thorofare, N.J.: 1995). 2013;**29**(9):590-595

[15] Montés-Micó R, Rodríguez-Galietero A, Alió JL.

Femtosecond laser versus mechanical keratome LASIK for myopia. Ophthalmology. 2007;**114**(1):62-68

[16] Chen X, Yu Y, Song X, Zhu Y, Wang W, Yao K. Clinical outcomes of femtosecond laser-assisted cataract surgery versus conventional phacoemulsification surgery for hard nuclear cataracts. Journal of Cataract and Refractive Surgery. 2017;**43**(4):486-491

[17] Mariacher S, Ebner M, Seuthe A-M, Januschowski K, Ivanescu C, Opitz N, et al. Femtosecond laser-assisted cataract surgery: First clinical results with special regard to central corneal thickness, endothelial cell count, and aqueous flare levels. Journal of Cataract and Refractive Surgery. 2016;**42**(8):1151-1156

[18] Alió JL, Abdou AA, Puente AA, Zato MA, Nagy Z. Femtosecond laser cataract surgery: Updates on technologies and outcomes. Journal of Refractive Surgery (Thorofare, N.J.: 1995). 2014;**30**(6):420-427

[19] Nagy ZZ, Takacs AI, Filkorn T, Kránitz K, Gyenes A, Juhász É, et al. Complications of femtosecond laser-assisted cataract surgery. Journal of Cataract and Refractive Surgery. 2014;**40**(1):20-28

[20] Mayer WJ, Klaproth OK, Hengerer FH, Kohnen T. Impact of crystalline lens opacification on effective phacoemulsification time in femtosecond laser-assisted cataract surgery. American Journal of Ophthalmology. 2014;**157**(2):426-432.e1

[21] Zhang J, Zhou Y, Zheng Y, Liu Q, Zhai C, Wang Y. Effect of suction on macular and retinal nerve fiber layer thickness during femtosecond lenticule extraction and femtosecond laser-assisted laser in situ keratomileusis. Journal of Cataract and Refractive Surgery. 2014;**40**(12):1994-2001

[22] Kang M-J, Lee Y-E, Choi J-S, Joo C-K. Ideal parameters for femto-second laser-assisted anterior capsulotomy: Animal studies. PLoS One. 2018;**13**(1):e0190858

[23] Diakonis VF, Yesilirmak N, Cabot F, Kankariya VP, Kounis GA, Warren D, et al. Comparison of surgically induced astigmatism between femtosecond laser and manual clear corneal incisions for cataract surgery. Journal of Cataract and Refractive Surgery. 2015;**41**(10):2075-2080

[24] Hoffmann PC, Hütz WW. Analysis of biometry and prevalence data for corneal astigmatism in 23,239 eyes. Journal of Cataract and Refractive Surgery. 2010;**36**(9):1479-1485

[25] Baharozian CJ, Song C, Hatch KM, Talamo JH. A novel nomogram for the treatment of astigmatism with femtosecond-laser arcuate incisions at the time of cataract surgery. Clinical Ophthalmology (Auckland, N.Z.). 2017 13;**11**:1841-1848

[26] Bali SJ, Hodge C, Lawless M, Roberts TV, Sutton G. Early experience with the femtosecond laser for cataract surgery. Ophthalmology. 2012;**119**(5):891-899

[27] Malyugin B, Sobolev N, Arbisser LB, Anisimova N. Combined use of an iris hook and pupil expansion ring for femtosecond laser-assisted cataract surgery in patients with cataracts complicated by insufficient mydriasis and an ectopic pupil. Journal of Cataract and Refractive Surgery. 2016;**42**(8):1112-1118

[28] Gupta PC, Ram J. Femtosecond laser–assisted cataract surgery in complex cases. Journal of Cataract and Refractive Surgery. 2016;**42**(11):1693

[29] Scott WJ, Tauber S, Gessler JA, Ohly JG, Owsiak RR, Eck CD. Comparison of vitreous loss rates

between manual phacoemulsification and femtosecond laser-assisted cataract surgery. Journal of Cataract and Refractive Surgery. 2016;**42**(7):1003-1008

[30] Sutton G, Bali SJ, Hodge C. Femtosecond cataract surgery: Transitioning to laser cataract. Current Opinion in Ophthalmology. 2013;**24**(1):3-8

[31] Ye Z, Li Z, He S. A meta-analysis comparing postoperative complications and outcomes of femtosecond laser-assisted cataract surgery versus conventional phacoemulsification for cataract. Journal of Ophthalmology. 2017;**2017**:3849152

[32] Popovic M, Campos-Möller X, Schlenker MB, Ahmed IIK. Efficacy and safety of femtosecond laser-assisted cataract surgery compared with manual cataract surgery: A meta-analysis of 14567 eyes. Ophthalmology. 2016;**123**(10):2113-2126

[33] Abell RG, Kerr NM, Howie AR, Mustaffa Kamal MAA, Allen PL, Vote BJ. Effect of femtosecond laser-assisted cataract surgery on the corneal endothelium. Journal of Cataract and Refractive Surgery. 2014;**40**(11):1777-1783

[34] Conrad-Hengerer I, Sheikh MA, Hengerer FH, Schultz T, Dick HB. Comparison of visual recovery and refractive stability between femtosecond laser–assisted cataract surgery and standard phacoemulsification: Six-month follow-up. Journal of Cataract and Refractive Surgery. 2015;**41**(7):1356-1364

[35] Jun JH, Yoo Y-S, Lim SA, Joo C-K. Effects of topical ketorolac tromethamine 0.45% on intraoperative miosis and prostaglandin E2 release during femtosecond laser-assisted cataract surgery. Journal of Cataract and Refractive Surgery. 2017;**43**(4):492-497

[36] Jun JH, Hwang KY, Chang SD, Joo C-K. Pupil-size alterations induced by photodisruption during femtosecond laser–assisted cataract surgery. Journal of Cataract and Refractive Surgery. 2015;**41**(2):278-285

[37] Panthier C, Costantini F, Rigal-Sastourné JC, Brézin A, Mehanna C, Guedj M, et al. Change of capsulotomy over 1 year in femtosecond laser-assisted cataract surgery and its impact on visual quality. Journal of Refractive Surgery (Thorofare, N.J.: 1995). 2017;**33**(1):44-49

[38] Taravella MJ, Meghpara B, Frank G, Gensheimer W, Davidson R. Femtosecond laser–assisted cataract surgery in complex cases. Journal of Cataract and Refractive Surgery. 2016;**42**(6):813-816

[39] Baig NB, Cheng GPM, Lam JKM, Jhanji V, Chong KKL, Woo VCP, et al. Intraocular pressure profiles during femtosecond laser-assisted cataract surgery. Journal of Cataract and Refractive Surgery. 2014;**40**(11):1784-1789

[40] Tran DB, Vargas V, Potvin R. Neodymium:YAG capsulotomy rates associated with femtosecond laser-assisted versus manual cataract surgery. Journal of Cataract and Refractive Surgery. 2016;**42**(10):1470-1476

[41] Bartlett JD, Miller KM. The economics of femtosecond laser-assisted cataract surgery. Current Opinion in Ophthalmology. 2016;**27**(1):76-81

[42] Donaldson KE, Braga-Mele R, Cabot F, Davidson R, Dhaliwal DK, Hamilton R, et al. Femtosecond laser-assisted cataract surgery. Journal of Cataract and Refractive Surgery. 2013;**39**(11):1753-1763

Chapter 3

Keratoconus Treatment Toolbox: An Update

Vatookarn Roongpoovapatr, Mohamed Abou Shousha and Puwat Charukamnoetkanok

Abstract

Keratoconus is a bilateral, asymmetric, progressive disease of the cornea which can lead to visual impairment and blindness as irregular astigmatism increases and corneal scar occurs. Currently, many methods are available for a treatment of keratoconus. The treatment can help enhance visual rehabilitation and prevent progression in keratoconus patients. The treatment options included non-surgical and surgical managements. This review offers a summary of the current and emerging treatment options for keratoconus- eyeglasses, contact lens, corneal collagen cross-linking (CXL), CXL Plus, intrastromal corneal ring segment (ICRS), Corneal Allogenic Intrastromal Ring Segments (CAIRS), Penetrating Keratoplasty (PK), Deep Anterior Lamellar Keratoplasty (DALK), Bowman layer transplantation (BL transplantation) and gene therapy.

Keywords: corneal collagen cross-linking, CXL, CXL Plus, intrastromal corneal ring segment, ICRS, PK, DALK, Bowman layer transplantation

1. Introduction

Keratoconus is a bilateral, asymmetric, progressive ectatic disease of the cornea characterized by progressive corneal thinning which can lead to visual impairment and blindness as corneal protrusion progresses, irregular astigmatism increases and corneal scar occurs [1]. Keratoconus is often under the radar because of decreased awareness, underdiagnosis and undertreatment. The exact pathological mechanism remains unknown, but both genetic and environmental factors may contribute to development and progression of this disease [2]. The reported evidences of pathogenesis of keratoconus include histochemistry, biomechanics, enzymology, proteomics, and molecular genetics [2]. The disease process starts with fragmentation of the epithelial basement membrane, fibrillation of Bowman's membrane and anterior stroma [3]. Bowman's membrane breakage occurs later together with epithelial abnormality resulting in proteolytic enzymes release that weakens corneal stromal collagen and stromal thinning [3]. The reported prevalence of keratoconus varies between countries and ethnicities, in which Asian is higher than Caucasian about 4.4 to 7.5 times [4, 5]. The prevalence is ranged from 0.3 in 100, 000 to 2300 in 100,000 in Russia and India respectively [6]. However, the prevalence may be higher in tertiary eye care center or refractive surgery center [7]. Keratoconus is more common in men than women, although both gender are affected [5]. The onset of symptoms usually presents during adolescent and may progress until the 30s. Keratoconus is associated with eye rubbing such as in allergic conjunctivitis, floppy eyelid syndrome, obstructive sleep apnea, Down's syndrome and Leber congenital amaurosis [1, 8–10]. Genetic predisposition accounts for an increased risk of keratoconus in patient that has a positive family history about 15 to 67 times [11].

2. Terminology and staging

Nowadays, there remain many controversies regarding disease definition, diagnosis, and management of keratoconus. Keratoconus is usually a bilateral disease in which the normal contralateral eye is believed to be in the preclinical stage of keratoconus with different terms such as subclinical keratoconus, keratoconus suspect, forme fruste keratoconus [12]. Despite the advancement of the investigations for the diagnosis of keratoconus and subclinical keratoconus, there are no definitive criteria for discriminating subclinical keratoconus from normal cornea currently [13]. The detection of keratoconus and subclinical keratoconus is crucial to prevent ectasia after refractive surgery. Moreover, some treatment modalities such as corneal collagen crosslinking can prevent vision loss in keratoconus if implement in the early stage of the disease [14]. The early stage symptoms may manifest as reduced vision, fluctuation of vision, progressive myopia and astigmatism, increasing higher order aberrations [4, 15]. When the disease progresses into an advance stage, there is a severe visual loss from high myopia, irregular astigmatism and corneal scarring.

The following criteria are mandatory to diagnose keratoconus- abnormal posterior elevation, abnormal corneal thickness distribution and clinical non-inflammatory corneal thinning [10]. However, there is no clinically adequate classification system for keratoconus currently. One of the most popular grading systems is Amsler-Krumeich classification system which classified severity of diseases based on the amount of myopia and astigmatism, corneal thickness or scarring and central keratometry readings [16, 17]. However, Amsler-Krumeich classification system is considered as outdated because it relies on "old" indices (corneal steepness, refractive change, the presence of scarring), and fails to address disease impact [18]. Nowadays, other alternate classification systems are growing in number such as Shabayek-Alio system which is based on corneal higher aberrations and the keratoconus severity score (KSS) which considers average corneal power and root mean square (RMS) [19, 20]. The "ABCD grading system" that incorporates anterior and posterior corneal curvature, thinnest pachymetric values based on the thinnest point and distant visual acuity may better reflects the anatomical change than some previous classification that uses pachymetric value based on apical measurement [21]. In routine clinical practice, the term "advanced keratoconus" usually apply to any case with unacceptably poor spectacle distance vision and contact lens intolerance [18].

3. Diagnosis

The keratoconus diagnosis is bases on the history and clinical examination. However, the investigations are very useful to augment the clinical examination and detect the early stage of disease. Moreover, the accurate diagnosis and early detection of keratoconus in essential in this era which laser refractive surgery has increased markedly. Failure to detect keratoconus and subclinical keratoconus can lead to ectasia after refractive surgery [22]. Corneal topography is the primary diagnostic tool for keratoconus detection. However, corneal topography is not a faultless method and therefore other diagnostic tools such as corneal pachymetry to characterize the corneal thinning and aberrometry to characterize degradation of the corneal optics should be used as complimentary techniques [22]. Corneal tomography which based on rotating Scheimpflug camera, such as Pentacam, Galilei, or Sirius systems, provide the topographic, pachymetric, and aberrometric information simultaneously as their use is adequate enough for the keratoconus detection [12, 22]. Currently, OCT technology is being used to differentiate between eye with keratoconus and normal eye because it can provide accurate pachymetric characterization, define epithelial thickness irregularity and asymmetry that present in keratoconus [7, 23]. By analyzing the biomechanical properties of the cornea that may precede the anatomical change, the Ocular Response Analyzer and Corvis systems can provide good diagnostic accuracy [22]. Analysis of the Corneal Microstructure change in keratoconic eye from confocal microscopy such as reducing corneal nerve fiber density and nerve fiber length, reducing keratocyte density, increasing corneal stromal nerve thickness, may be useful in detecting structural changes occurring before manifestation of topographic signs [22, 24]. A combination of multiple imaging modalities, including corneal topography, corneal tomography, Scheimpflug imaging, anterior segment optical coherence tomography, and in vivo confocal microscopy will enhance early keratoconus detection. Modalities during investigations but show promise include polarization-sensitive optical coherence tomography, Brillouin microscopy, and atomic force microscopy [25].

4. Disease progression

Keratoconus progression detection is a critical issue because the treatment nomograms have been proposed based on the grading system and ectasia progression [15, 22]. Moreover, the disease progression is differed considerably among individual. The younger the patients are, the higher their risk for rapid progression [26]. Currently, there is no global consensus of ectasia progression. The Group of Panelists for the Global Delphi Panel of Keratoconus and Ectatic Diseases had defined the definition of "ectasia progression" as a consistent change overtime in at least 2 of the following parameters where the magnitude of the change is above the normal noise of the testing system:

1. Steepening of the anterior corneal surface.

2. Steepening of the posterior corneal surface.

3. Thinning and/or an increase in the rate of corneal thickness change from the periphery to the thinnest point" [10].

Various clinical studies have used different parameters to define disease progression. The most important parameters include: [27, 28]

1. An increase in maximum corneal refractive power (K_{max}) by more than 1 diopter (D) within 1 year

2. An increase in (corneal) myopia by more than 3 D or astigmatism by more than 1.5 D within 12 months

3. An increase in mean corneal refractive power by more than 1.5 D within 12 months

4. A reduction in minimal corneal thickness of more than 5% within 12 months.

The regular topographic/tomographic check-ups can identify keratoconus progression. Regarding the examination intervals, the individual risk profiles need to be taken into consideration. The risk factors that should be considered include eye rubbing, ocular allergies, young age, steep corneal curvature gradient, high astigmatism, marked visual loss, documented progression in the fellow eye, atopic dermatitis or Down's syndrome [28]. In children, keratoconus tends to be more severe and progress faster requiring closer follow-up intervals [26]. The patient with low risks can be monitored less frequently than the one with high risks. Keratoconus progression is often associated with a decrease in best spectacle-corrected visual acuity (BSCVA), however, a change in both uncorrected visual acuity and BSCVA is not required to document progression [10].

5. Treatment

The important goals of keratoconus management are stopping disease progression and visual rehabilitation [10]. In cases of ocular allergies, patients should be treated with topical antiallergy and lubricants and should be instructed to avoid eye rubbing to halt disease progression. Corneal collagen crosslinking is a promising procedure to stop disease progression with minimal side effects [29]. For the visual rehabilitation, several treatment options corresponding to keratoconus grading have been established. Keratoconus can be treated by both nonsurgical and surgical approaches depend on severity and progression of the disease [15]. The keratoconus treatment toolbox is listed as in **Table 1**.

Nonsurgical treatments	Surgical treatments
• **Glasses** • **Contact lens (CL)** Soft CL; toric, non-toric Rigid CL; RGP Hybrid lenses, Piggyback lens (PBCL) Miniscleral Semiscleral Scleral lenses	• **Corneal collagen cross-linking (CXL)** Standard CXL Epi-on CXL Accelerated CXL CXL Plus CXL + TG-PRK CXL + ICRS CXL + TG- PRK + phakic IOLS CXL + ICRS + phakic IOLS CXL in thin cornea • **Intrastromal corneal ring segments (ICRS)** • **Corneal transplantation** Penetrating keratoplasty (PK) Deep Anterior Lamellar Keratoplasty (DALK) Bowman layer transplantation

RGP = Rigid gas permeable contact lens, IOL = intraocular lenses, PBCL = Piggyback lens, TG-PRK = Topo guided-Photo Refractive Keratectomy.

Table 1.
The keratoconus treatment toolbox.

5.1 Nonsurgical treatment

A nonsurgical treatment of keratoconus is spectacles and contact lens. For early stage of disease, those who achieve visual acuity 20/40 or better, spectacles can provide acceptable vision [15]. A toric soft contact lens also provides satisfactory vision for correcting myopia and regular astigmatism in early keratoconus. However, as the diseases progress, spectacles or soft contact lens may not provide acceptable vision because of the higher- order aberrations, in particular vertical coma was increased [30]. Therefore, other special lens such as rigid gas permeable (RGP) contact lens, hybrid lenses, piggy back, miniscleral lens, semiscleral lens or scleral lenses are needed to provide satisfactory vision [31]. The ultimate goal of fitting contact lens in keratoconus is to improve visual acuity without compromise ocular health. However, contact lens use does not slow or stop progression of the disease. In keratoconus, the cone is steeper but the cornea beyond the cone is flatter. In mild keratoconus, traditional RGP lens can provide an ideal fit. However, as the disease progress into advanced stages, it becomes difficult to achieve an ideal fit but compromised fit which is not damage to the ocular surface is acceptable. High oxygen transmissibility lens should be selected to prevent hypoxic-related corneal changes [31].

The type of contact lens selection is based on manifest refraction, degree of keratoconus, and morphology of the cone [31]. Corneal topography can aid in addressing the severity and morphology of the cone. Buxton et al. have classified keratoconus based on keratometry values (K) at the apex of the cone: mild if K is less than 45 D, moderate if K is between 45 and 52 D, advanced if K is more than 52 D and severe if K is more than 62 D [32]. The morphology of the cone is classifed as the following [33].

- nipple cone: small, paracentral, steeper located inferiorly or inferonasally
- oval cone: inferiorly or inferotemporally steeper cornea
- globus cone: overall steeper cornea, involves more than three forth of the cornea up to limbus

The three essential parameters in contact lens fitting are power, diameter, and base curve of contact lens.

- Power: Low minus for mild keratoconus, high minus for severe keratoconus
- Base curve: Flatter base curve for mild keratoconus, steeper base curve for severe keratoconus
- Diameter: Based on the cone location, its size and steepness, nipple has a small diameter, usually start with a small diameter such as 8.7 mm, oval cone needs larger diameter lens, globus cone or severe apical displacement need large diameter contact lens.

A contact lens type is selected based on the manifest refraction and the degree of keratoconus. The contact lens of choice for keratoconus patients is RGP lens. However, if the patients develop intolerance or discomfort, customized soft toric contact lens, PBCL, hybrid lens or scleral lens can be considered. The indications, advantages and disadvantages of each contact lens type are summarized as in **Table 2** [30, 31, 34]. Fitting contact lens in keratoconus can improve vision and

Contact lens types	Indication	Advantages	Disadvantages
Soft/ Soft toric	• For mild KC • High myopia associated with KC • Intolerance/ discomfort with RGP • Prior to PBCL	• Comfort	• Cannot correct irregular astigmatism
RGP	• First lens of choice for KC patient	• First lens of choice for visual improvement • Can correct irregular astigmatism	• Less comfortable than other CLs • Need lens adaptation • Inappropriate fitting can compromise ocular health • May associated with increase keratoconus progression [35]
Hybrid lens	• RGP intolerance • Inability to obtain optimal RGP fitting • Poor RGP centering • Reduced wearing time with RGP	Comfort	• Risk of hypoxia, corneal edema, neovascularization
Piggyback lens (PBCL)	• Discomfort or RGP intolerance • Irregular cornea where RGP lens fitting are not possible • (unstable RGP on the eye, popping out of lens • 3 and 9 o' clock staining with RGP • Corneal scarring	Comfort	• Lost RGP • GPC • Risk of hypoxia, corneal edema, neovascularization • Punctate keratitis • Difficult handling and maintaining
Scleral lens	• All options fail to improve vision • Inability to get an optimum fit with RGP • RGP intolerance • 3 and 9 o' clock staining with RGP • Vascularization with PBCL • Advanced keratoconus • Corneal scarring • Associated ocular diseases	• Comfort • Stable VA • Delays or obviates the need for keratoplasty	• Difficult in care regimen (require different removal and insertion technique) • Contraindicate in corneal edema, acute hydrops, post filtration surgery

RGP = Rigid gas permeable, Hybrid lens = rigid lens in the center and a soft skirt in the periphery, PBCL = Piggy back lens (RGP lens sitting on top of a soft contact lens) KC = keratoconus, GPC = giant papillary conjunctivitis, VA = visual acuity.

Table 2.
Contact lens in keratoconus (KC).

delay the need for keratoplasty. Moreover, contact lens in keratoconus patient also have a role in correcting residual refractive error after Corneal collagen cross-linking (CXL), after Intrastromal corneal ring segments (ICRS) or post-keratoplasty [31].

5.2 Surgical treatment

Even though the specialized imaging device can provide grading scheme of keratoconus, for practical purposes, the term "advanced keratoconus" may apply to any cases that have unacceptably poor spectacle distance vision and contact lens intolerance. As the diseases progress, spectacles or contact lens cannot provide acceptable vision. This group of patients requires a surgical management such as Corneal collagen cross-linking (CXL), Intrastromal corneal ring segments (ICRS), and Corneal transplantation to restore vision and/or stabilize progression of diseases.

The special considerations in surgical management of keratoconus are listed in **Table 3**.

5.2.1 Corneal collagen cross-linking (CXL)

Keratoconus typically progresses until the fourth decade, when most but not all, slows or stabilizes [36]. Corneal crosslinking (CXL) has been proposed as a new treatment modality to stop progression of keratoconus since the late 1990s [27]. Currently, CXL is the gold standard and only minimally invasive surgical procedure that halt the progression of keratoconus [27]. The indications for CXL are progressive keratoconus in adults and postoperative ectasia, central corneal thickness more than 400 μm, K_{max} 58 D or less [36, 38]. However, the procedure is not approved for stable keratoconus currently. CXL is the promising treatment that can prevent progressive visual loss due to disease evolution and delay invasive surgical procedures such as corneal transplantation. The mechanism of cornea strengthening is a photochemical reaction of corneal collagen by the Riboflavin as a photosensitizer in the photopolymerization process and ultraviolet A irradiation (UVA). The interaction between Riboflavin and UVA can increases the formation of intrafibrillar and interfibrillar carbonyl-based collagen covalent bonds [37].

The standard Dresden protocol was proposed as a treatment option for keratoconus by Wollensak et al. in 2003 [38]. This standard technique is conducted under topical anesthesia. The central corneal epithelium is removed followed by application of 0.1% riboflavin solution (0.1% riboflavin in 20% dextran solution) as a photosensitizer every 5 minutes for 30 minutes. Then the cornea is exposed to 370 nm UVA with an irradiance of 3 mW/cm^2 or 5.4 J/cm^2, during which time riboflavin solution is re-applied every 5 minutes. After the treatment, topical antibiotics eye drops are applied and bandage contact lens placed upon the eye [38]. Although this standard protocol has been proven to be an effective procedure to halt keratoconus progression [39], it is a time-consuming procedure, may create patient discomfort and has post-operative complications related to corneal abrasion. The reported complications in association with CXL include corneal haze, corneal infection, corneal edema, and corneal melting. Adverse effects are common but mostly transient and of low clinical significance [40]. However, anterior corneal stromal haze is a typical postoperative finding that often occurs in the first month after treatment and typically resolves after 12 to 20 weeks [41]. The posterior aspect of this haze is an indistinct hyperreflective demarcation line seen in the mid stroma that represents the depth of CXL [37]. Two trends have emerged to modify the standard Dresden protocol. The first is a tendency to shorten treatment times [42]. Alternative treatment protocols with different formulations of riboflavin solution

Considerations	Details
Corneal thickness (Corneal thinness)	• **CXL**: CCT > 400 μm can use standard Dresden protocol CCT < 400 μm • Hypotonic riboflavin solution Epi-on CXL* • Pachymetry-guided epithelial debridement Decreasing the UVA irradiance dose • Reducing the duration of riboflavin soaking Increasing the riboflavin concentration or a combination of the above • **ICRS**: minimum corneal thickness at the site of their insertion and along the length of their path >400 μm • **Bowman layer transplantation**: do not affect • **DALK**: Prefer Melles manual dissection than Anwar "big-bubble" technique • **PK**: not suitable for significant peripheral thinning DALK or modified procedure "tuck-in lamellar keratoplasty" may be preferable
Kmax	• **CXL**: risk of failure, continue progression in $K_{max>}$ 58 D, increase risk of losing vision in $K_{max>}$ 55 D • **ICRS**: associated with poorer visual outcomes and more complications in $K_{max>}$ 58 D • **Bowman layer transplantation**: do not affect • **DALK**: central curvatures >60 diopters (D) may experience worse outcomes • **PK**: do not affect
Preoperative BCVA	• **CXL, ICRS, Bowman layer transplantation**: rarely do the visual gain exceed 1 0r 2 lines • **DALK or PK**: extremely poor vision
Endothelial health	• **CXL**: risks of endothelial damage if CCT < 400 μm • **ICRS, Bowman layer transplantation, DALK**: No or mild endothelial dystrophy • **PK**: advanced KC and a failed endothelium
Lens status	• **CXL, ICRS, Bowman layer transplantation**: not promote cataractogenesis, preferable options for phakic eyes • **DALK**: No/less cataractogenesis than PK • **PK**: cataractogenesis, may be the least desirable option for phakic eyes
Patient age (Pediatric)	• **CXL**: modest corneal flattening effect, mild visual benefit without any additional complications, smaller gain and less durable than adults • **ICRS**: approved for age > 18 years (worldwide), 21 years in US, no difference between visual outcome or corneal topography between different age groups • **Bowman layer transplantation**: extraocular procedure, one of the safest options • **DALK**: similar outcomes with adults • **PK**: outcomes are slightly worse, principally attributable to higher rates of graft rejection, failure

Considerations	Details
Ability to cooperate (Mental disability)	• **CXL**: risk of postoperative complications, only patients capable of reliable cooperation, with good family support • **ICRS**: less risky and fewer postoperative requirements than CXL, DALK, PK but aware of ICRS stem from migration/ superficialization from eye rubbing • **Bowman layer transplantation**: less risky and fewer postoperative requirements than CXL, DALK, PK • **DALK**: may be preferred over PK • **PK**: worse outcomes from higher incidence of postoperative complications
Pre-existing corneal scarring (previous hydrops)	• **CXL**: may be less successful, cannot replace corneal scar then central corneal scar is a relative contraindication • **ICRS, Bowman layer transplantation**: central corneal scar is a contraindication, may arrest disease progression and permit continued CL wear in non- visually disabling scarring • **DALK**: may be preferred over PK, prefer Melles manual dissection, Anwar "big-bubble" technique is contraindicated • **PK**: outcomes tend to be worse (not be considered mandatory to replace endothelium)

*CCT = central corneal thicknesses, Epi-on CXL = Epithelium-On Corneal collagen cross-linking, ICRS = Intrastromal corneal ring segments, DALK = Deep Anterior Lamellar Keratoplasty, PK = Penetrating keratoplasty, D = diopter, KC = keratoconus, K_{max} = Maximal corneal steepness, BCVA = best corrected visual acuity. Adapted from Surv Ophthalmol. 2015 Sep;60(5):459–80. [18] J Cataract Refract Surg. 2015 Apr;41(4):842–72 [37]. *currently little to recommend UV-CXL in corneas thinner than 400 μm [18] .*

Table 3.
Special considerations in surgical management of keratoconus.

and delivery methods by altered UV exposures have been proposed. These newer techniques can shorten duration times, reduce patient discomfort, and minimize postoperative complications. The second trend is "epi-on" approach, such that the epithelium remains intact during CXL. These modifications were described in the following sections.

5.2.1.1 Accelerated CXL (ACXL)

According to Bunsen- Roscoe law of photochemical reciprocity, which states that "the same photochemical effect can be achieved with a reduced irradiation interval provided the total energy level is kept constant through a corresponding increase in irradiation intensity" [37]. ACXL is a modified CXL technique that increase the intensity of ultraviolet A (UV-A) irradiation and shortening the exposure time without altering the total energy delivered. Currently commercial devices now offer ultrafast settings such as 43 mW/cm^2 for 2 minutes [42]. Using this setting, would achieve the standard Dresden protocol energy dose of 3.4 J or a radiant exposure of 5.4 J/cm^2 within 2 minutes [42]. However, it ignores the requirement of oxygen in the CXL reaction, the time needed for oxygen replenishment, and potential physical damage due to higher irradiance [36]. The reduced efficacy of ACXL is believed to be due to depletion of oxygen in these high-fluence treatments [43]. The efficacy, safety, and treatment protocols of accelerated CXL are still being investigated and in evolution.

5.2.1.2 Epi-on CXL/transepithelial CXL

Due to the epithelial debridement is a major contributor to the postoperative complications of CXL, such as infective keratitis and an abnormal wound-healing response [37]. This issue has perpetuated interest in epithelium-on technique. Epi-on CXL has less discomfort to the patient and reduces postoperative complications [43]. This CXL technique has low complication rate, 0% to 3.9% of the patients has only transient haze [37]. According to the hydrophilic property of riboflavin solution, the penetration through the intact hydrophobic corneal epithelium is difficult. The standard formulations show minimal penetration through intact epithelium. The modifications by adding various additives, such as benzalkonium chloride, topical anesthetic, tris(hydroxymethyl) aminomethane (trometamol), sodium ethylenediaminetetraacetic acid, have been proposed to improve epithelial permeability to riboflavin [36]. Riboflavin penetration can be improved by increased riboflavin concentration and iontophoresis [36]. Since even the low amount of riboflavin surface films will markedly block UV-A transmission, transepithelial formulations are often rinsed from epithelial surface before irradiation [36]. The iontophoretic delivery system uses of mild electrical current for delivering riboflavin through the epithelium [36]. It allows greater and deeper riboflavin penetration in the corneal stroma than the conventional epithelium-on technique. Overall, the effectiveness of transepithelial techniques has been disappointing [27]. Epi-on CXL has limited keratocyte apoptosis, shallower demarcation line and less biomechanical rigidity than standard epi-off CXL [37]. In general, better outcomes can be achieved by standard epithelium off technique and epi-on CXL have resulted in progression of the disease after treatment [36, 44]. However, recent research with innovative transepithelial CXL system achieved 4-fold higher corneal stromal concentrations of riboflavin than commercially available epi-on CXL system, and this level is theoretically adequate for effective CXL [44].

5.2.1.3 Pulsed-light accelerated CXL (PLA-CXL)

Due to the presence of oxygen is required for CXL, but high-exposure doses of UVA light cause a decrease in the oxygen concentration rapidly [45]. The recent technique has focused on pulsing the UVA light with "on" and "off" periods to increase the efficacy of CXL treatment by replenishing the consumed oxygen [46]. This technique is an effective treatment modality to stop progression in progressive keratoconus but regresses some of the cases [46].

5.2.1.4 CXL plus

Despite the fact that CXL can halt the progression of keratoconus and provide corneal stability, functional visual acuity remains a problem [47]. Recent data from the systematic review disclosed that conventional epi-off CXL can flattening cornea 2 D approximately and improving visual acuity 2 lines or 10 letters on average [48]. CXL normalizes the corneal shape by changing the physical properties of the cornea, resulting in reduction of all corneal aberrations, high order and low order. The improvement in uncorrected distance visual acuity (UDVA) and corrected distance visual acuity (CDVA) are related to improvement in the total corneal aberrations and only high-order aberrations respectively [49].

In order to address this issue, CXL can be performed alone or in combination with topo guided photorefractive keratectomy (PRK), ICRS, phakic IOLS or Topo guided PRK plus ICRS for better improvement of visual acuity [15].

- CXL + Topo guided PRK

Kanellopoulos et al. reported the first case of topography-guided PRK performed 1 year after CXL for treatment of keratoconus and showed visual acuity improvement [50]. On the contrary, the Athens protocol which combines accelerated UV-CXL with same-day photorefractive keratectomy (PRK) was more effective with improvement in UDVA and CDVA of 20/45 or better (2.25 logMAR) was founded in 83% of patients at last follow up [51]. However, this study was conducted in post-LASIK ectasia [51]. Same-day simultaneous topography guided PRK CXL in progressive keratoconus appears to be superior to sequential CXL with later PRK (6 months later) in the aspect of UCVA, BSCVA, spherical equivalent (SE) and mean reduction in K [52]. This combined technique also prevents regression of keratoconus and reduce the risk of keratectasia and might be suitable for eyes requiring improvements in irregular astigmatisms but still have good CDVA [47, 53].

- CXL + ICRS

The CXL can be performed before, simultaneously or after the ICRS. The advantage of performing the CXL first is slowing the progression of the keratoconus and selects the best alternative way to treat the residual refractive error [54]. The recent systematic review and meta-analysis demonstrated that simultaneous ICRS implantation and CXL may provide better outcomes in term of refraction and keratometry. However, UDVA, BCVA and cylindrical refractive error were similar between combined technique and staged procedure [55]. The combined procedure of CXL plus ICRS implantation appears safe and efficacious for the treatment of progressive keratoconus with significant improvements in visual acuity, keratometry values, and refractive error [54]. This technique might be effective for eyes with more irregular astigmatism and worse CDVA [53].

- CXL + Topo guided PRK + phakic IOLS

The simultaneous topography-guided photorefractive keratectomy (PRK) and crosslinking (Athens protocol) followed by phakic intraocular lens (IOL) implantation 2–4 months later for managing keratoconus improved and stabilized visual performance in patients with keratoconus. The K_{mean}, SE, UDVA, CDVA improved significantly. At last follow-up, all eyes could achieve CDVA of 0.3 or better [56].

- CXL + ICRS+ + phakic IOLS

Three steps treatment of keratoconus by ICRS implantation, CXL and phakic IOLS significantly improve UDVA, CDVA, higher order aberrations and corneal shape in moderate to severe keratoconus [57]. Moreover, keratometry (K_{steep}, K_{flat}, K_{max}) and refraction (sphere, SE, but not cylinder) were also improved [58]. The time interval between ICRS implantation and CXL was 4–6 weeks and ICL implantation was performed 6–8 months after CXL [57, 58].

5.2.1.5 CXL in thin cornea

The 0.1% riboflavin in 20% dextran solution is used in original Dresden protocol. Only the anterior 300 μm of stroma can be treated [38, 59]. This standard technique requires corneal pachymetry more than 400 μm after de-epithelization to decrease complications such as corneal stromal scar and corneal endothelial cytotoxicity [47, 60]. In order to combat this issue, there are various modifications to the conventional CXL protocol for CXL in thin cornea. These modifications include hypoosmolar riboflavin, transepithelial CXL, iontophoresis-assisted CXL, Customized epithelial debridement technique, Lenticule-assisted CXL, contact-lens- assisted CXL (CACXL) and individualized corneal CXL [60–67].

Hypoosmolar riboflavin has lower colloidal pressure (310 mOsmol/L vs. 402.7 mOsmol/L in isotonic riboflavin) that causes stromal swelling to double its thickness where stromal bed is less than 400 μm [60]. However, the efficacy of CXL using hypoosmolar riboflavin was lower than traditional CXL with isotonic riboflavin. The possible theory to explain is that in hydrated corneas (using hypoosmolar riboflavin) concentration of collagen fibrils is decreased, hence fewer collagen fibrils are available for CXL [60, 61]. By changing the osmolarity of the riboflavin solution, while maintaining the concentration at 0.1%, probably does not alter the final riboflavin concentration in the cornea. On the contrary, modifying other parameters to obtain a more shallow depth of treatment; ie, the intensity of the UVA light, the duration of treatment, or the intensity of riboflavin concentration will alter the final riboflavin concentration in the cornea and require new dose–response assays [61]. Unfortunately, these modified techniques have not yet distinguished themselves as more effective than any other in terms of topographic or visual outcomes.

Despite the fact that CXL has a promising clinical outcomes, risk factors for ongoing ectasia include the application of isotonic riboflavin solution to thicken a thin cornea prior to treatment, corneas steeper than 58 D and age > 35 years [18, 68]. The most frequent definition of treatment failure is the continual progression of keratoconus with an enhancement of K_{max} reading of 1.0 D 0r 1.5 D over the preoperative value [40, 47]. The outcomes of different CXL techniques are listed as in **Table 4**.

5.2.2 Intrastromal corneal ring segments (ICRS)

Intrastromal corneal ring segments (ICRS) were FDA-approved in 1999 for the treatment of low myopia. ICRS implantation causes displacement of the collagen fibers resulting in flattening of the central cornea and tissue adjacent to the ring is displaced forward [37]. ICRS are segments of polymethylmethacrylate (PMMA) plastic available in numerous arc-lengths, thicknesses, and designs. Five types of ICRS are available for keratoconus: 1) Intacs (Addition technology Inc.) 2) Intacs SK (Addition technology Inc.), 3) Ferrara Rings (Ferrara ophthalmics) and 4) Keraring (Mediphacos).5). MyoRing (Dioptex, GmbH, Linz, Austria). The devices are inserted into stromal tunnels that may be created manually using a corkscrew blade or femtosecond laser with no difference in results (except that channels tend to be slightly shallower when created manually and more often decentered when created by laser) [37]. The objective of ICRS implantation is to improve visual and topographic outcomes and restoration of contact lens tolerance [15, 18, 37]. Maximal flattening effect occurs with segments at 60–79% corneal thickness. Shallower than 60%, the effect may be lessened and can induced ocular surface complications. On the contrary, deeper than 80%, there may have no topographic effect [88]. The outcome achieved is directly proportional to the thickness of the ICRS and inversely proportional to its diameter [37]. ICRS can be used alone or used in combination with other treatment options such as CXL for stabilizing disease progression [15]. The outcomes of ICRS are listed as in **Table 4**.

Although, ICRS has good visual and topographic results, some complications have been reported. Intraoperative complications rate are low, but can occur and

DOI: http://dx.doi.org/10.5772/intechopen.94854

Treatment	Visual outcomes	Refractive outcomes	Topographic outcomes	Disease progression
Standard CXL	• VA either remains unchanged or improves by 1–2 lines [18, 38, 48, 49] • Corneas steeper than 58 D, no benefit in UDVA or BCVA [68]	• Small reduction in astigmatism <0.5 D [18, 70] • variable, unpredictable corneal astigmatic correction [71] • Sphere and cylinder was less negative, SE was more positive [49]	• Evening out of corneal parameters and a decline in overall surface variability [72] • Flattening Kmean and Kmax by 1–2 D [18, 38, 48, 49] • KFlat did not change [49] • advanced KC may demonstrate changes more frequently than mild disease [18] • Shortly after therapy, CCT may decline till 3 months but rebounds to baseline at 1 year [39]	• Stop progression > 90% -100% [68, 69, 74] • Stop progression 75% in pediatric patient [63]
Epi-on CXL/ Transepithelial CXL	• Improvement of UDVA and CDVA (logMAR) [49] • 3 months: 0.06 • 6 months: 0.17 12 months: 0.05 • 0.07 logMAR more improvement in CDVA than standard CXL [69] • Similar or lower UDVA with standard CXL [62, 69]	• No changes for the sphere, cylinder, and SE up to 12 months after CXL. [49] • Lower SE than standard CXL [69] • Similar increase refractive cylinder by 1.5 D and spherical refraction by 1.0 D as standard CXL [69]	• Less effective than standard CXL to reduce Kmax (mean difference = 1.05D) [62] • Kmax was reduced by 1.9–2.2 D,1 and 3 months after CXL but not later [49] • Stable Kmax (no flattening)or Kmax increase by 1.1 D [69, 73] • Kmin was reduced by 0.6 to 0.8 D, 1 and 3 months after CXL, and not later [49] • Ksteep was reduced by 1.9 and 1.2 D, 6 and 12 months, respectively, after CXL. [49] • Kavg was not changed [49] • Kflat, Ksteep increase slightly overtime (but decrease slightly overtime in standard CXL) [69] • Similar change in CCT with standard CXL or stable CCT [62, 69]	• 23–55% progression of the disease between 1 year- 3 years after treatment [44, 69, 73] • Stop progression 50% in pediatric patient with Iontophoretic Transepithelial CXL [63]

Treatment	Visual outcomes	Refractive outcomes	Topographic outcomes	Disease progression
Accelerated CXL	• No improvement in UDVA, BCVA [49] • UDVA and BCVA increased 1 Snellen line at 30 months [75] • Compare to standard CXL at 5 years [76] • Similar improve in UDVA by 0.08 logMAR • Similar improve in BCVA by 0.06 logMAR	• Similar reduction in astigmatism by 0.8–0.9 D, SE by 0.9 D when compare to standard CXL at 4 years [76] • Cylinder increased by 0.7 D 3 months after CXL, SE was more positive after 36 months by 1.07 D, sphere data were not reported [49]	• Similar reduction in K with standard CXL (Kflat, Ksteep Kmean by 1 D and Kmax by 1.7–2.2 D, at 5 years) [49, 76] • Greater reduction in Kmean than standard CXL [78] • Epi-on was less effective than Epi-off Accelerated CXL to reduce Kmean, Kmax [75] • Epi-on: stable CCT • Epi-off: decreased during the first 6 months and return to baseline at 1 year [75] • Less or similar corneal thinning than standard CXL [78, 79] • No significant changes in corneal topography parameters [49]	Conflicting findings [75]
Pulsed-Light Accelerated CXL	• CDVA improved by 0.11 logMAR at 6 months [49] • BCVA improved by 0.2 logMAR at 1 year [77] • BSCVA improved by 0.17 logMAR at 2 years [46]	• Corneal astigmatism increased by 0.3 D at 1 year [77]	• Kmax reduced by 1.2D at 1 year [77] • Flattening of Kmean and Kmax by 0.58 and 0.75 D at 2 years [46] • Thinnest corneal pachymetry reduced by 7–16 μm at 1–2 years [46, 77] • CCT reduced by 6 μm at 2 years	All eyes show stability of K_{max}, 30% show small increase in K_{max} at 12 months [77]

DOI: http://dx.doi.org/10.5772/intechopen.94854

Treatment	Visual outcomes	Refractive outcomes	Topographic outcomes	Disease progression
Intrastromal corneal ring segments (ICRS)	• Improve 1–2 lines of BSCVA and BCVA • Newer segment designs such as INTACS SK and Kerarings, visual gains still rarely exceed 1–2 lines and may increase visual aberrations. [18] • 10% lost ≥1 line of UDVA, and 20% lost ≥1 line of BCVA [80]	• Sizable reduction in corneal astigmatism from 1 to 3 D • Significant changes between 6 and 12 months • Full refractive effect is not seen before 1 year postoperatively • Appears stable, at least through 10 years of follow-up [18]	• Standard INTACS reduce mean Ks by 3–5 D [18] • INTACS SK, Kerarings, Ferrara ring, and Myoring reduce mean Ks by 2–9 D (smaller internal diameters and are placed closer to the corneal center) [18]	Stop progression >90% for mild to moderate KC at 5 and 10 years [68, 80, 83]
Penetrating keratoplasty (PK)	• UDVA 20/50 to 20/100 [18] • BCVA 20/30 to 20/40 [18]	• Average astigmatism 3 to 5 D but may exceed 10 D [18] • 20% require refractive surgery after surgery [18] • Suture removal tends to result in large unpredictable swings in the amount of astigmatism	Donor button is • oversized 0.5 mm; mean K around 45.5 D • same-sized; mean K around 42.5 D [18]	Approximately 10% of eyes will display recurrent KC 20 years after PK; some diseased recipient cornea is left unremoved [84, 85]
Deep Anterior Lamellar Keratoplasty (DALK)	• Descematic DALK; Similar/better UDVA, BSCVA, BCVA to PK [18, 81] • Pre-descematic DALK; inferior visual results to PK • Fewer higher aberrations than PK [18]	• Same refractive outcomes or more myopia than PK [18, 82]	2 D steeper than if they had received a similarly sized PK [18]	NA

Treatment	Visual outcomes	Refractive outcomes	Topographic outcomes	Disease progression
Bowman layer transplantation	• BSCVA typically improves by 1–2 lines • BCVA usually remains unchanged [18]	• Slight hyperopic shift with no significant effect on corneal astigmatism [86, 87]	• Mean reduction in anterior simulated Ks 5 D • max corneal power 5 to 7 D • K max 8–9-D [86, 87] • Non- significantly increase CCT, thinnest pachymetry [86] • These topographic changes occur within the first post-operative month and appear stable through at least 2 years	• Stop progression • 90% [87]

CXL = Corneal collagen cross-linking, PRK = Photorefractive keratectomy, IOL = intraocular lenses, UDVA = Uncorrected Distance visual acuity, CDVA = Corrected Distance visual acuity, BCVA = Best Corrected Visual Acuity, BSCVA = Best Spectacles Corrected visual acuity, D = Diopter, SE = spherical equivalent.
Other than standard CXL, formulation of riboflavin solutions, riboflavin concentration, total UVA energy that was used for each study may be different.

Table 4.
Outcomes of surgical treatment of keratoconus.

usually relate to corneal tunnel creation such as insufficient tunnel depth, asymmetry or decentration, or Bowman's layer perforation [15]. The post-operative complications have been reported such as corneal neovascularization, keratitis, deposits around ring segment, corneal haze, halos, pain, corneal melting or edema, segment extrusion, visual fluctuation, and photophobia [15]. This procedure is reversible and not preclude from further surgeries such as CXL and/or corneal transplantation. Due to complications such as stromal necrosis, segment extrusion of synthetic ICRS material, corneal allogenic ICRS (CAIRS) combined with CXL has been reported. Instead of using PMMA to create segment, CAIRS is trephined from donor cornea. CAIRS were implanted into mid-depth corneal tunnel that was created by femtosecond laser, followed by ACXL [89]. This procedure has a promising result in term of improvement of UDVA by 2.79 lines, CDVA by 1.29 lines. Moreover, this procedure demonstrated improvement of SE, K_{max}, K_{steep} and topographic astigmatism and halt progression in all cases during follow period [89].

5.2.3 Corneal transplantation

Treatment options for advanced keratoconus that has corneal thickness less than 400 μm, K_{max} more than 58 D may be limited to corneal transplantation that can stabilize the cone and enable continued contact lens wear [86]. The keratoplasty techniques may be penetrating keratoplasty (PK), Deep Anterior Lamellar Keratoplasty (DALK) or Bowman layer transplantation.

5.2.3.1 Penetrating keratoplasty (PK)

Penetrating or lamellar keratoplasty techniques are used depending on the extent of corneal scarring [15]. PK provides long term good vision but has slow visual rehabilitation from residual astigmatism and anisometropia [15]. Both PK and DALK tend to worsen any existing ocular surface problems, as both involve surface incisions, injury of corneal nerves, placement of long-lasting sutures, and requiring post-operative topical corticosteroids [18]. Despite the facts that long term graft survival following PK for keratoconus is good, averaging 97% at 5 years, 90% at 10 years and 80% at 20–25 years, most of the patients with advanced KC are transplanted early in life, therefore it is more likely that more than one graft may be required over their lifetime ultimately [18].

5.2.3.2 Deep anterior lamellar keratoplasty (DALK)

The visual outcomes of BCVA, UDVA for DALK remains debated. The recent data from systematic review and meta-analysis demonstrated that the visual outcomes were worse [90] or better [81] than those for PK. The outcomes of DALK for keratoconus are better than PK [81] or equivalent [81] in terms of refractive error, astigmatism and rejection rate. Fifty percent of eyes may encounter Descemet membrane perforation which is the most significant intra-operative complications [18]. Other complications such as a double anterior chamber and persistent corneal edema have been reported. DALK may be less prone to secondary ocular hypertension because of their lower steroid requirement (owing to the smaller risk of rejection) [18]. Another advantage DALK is the lack of endothelial rejection because there is no endothelial defense reaction [15]. The reported rates of postoperative complications such as graft rejection, secondary glaucoma, complicated cataracts, and constant endothelial cell loss are lower with DALK than PK [15].

Classification* Disease progression	Management			
	Stage 1	Stage 2	Stage 3	Stage 4
Non- progressive	Spectacles	Spectacles		
	CL	CL	CL	CL
			CL intolerance	CL intolerance
	ICRS	ICRS		
			BL transplantation	BL transplantation
				DALK/PK
Progressive	Spectacles	Spectacles		
	CL	CL	CL	CL
			CL intolerance	CL intolerance
	CXL	CXL	CXL	
	ICRS	ICRS		
			BL transplantation	BL transplantation
				DALK/PK

Adapted from JAMA Ophthalmol. 2014 Apr 1;132(4):495–501.
The classification of keratoconus was based on Krumeich JH et al.A. Live-epikeratophakia for keratoconus. J Cataract Refract Surg. 1998 Apr;24(4):456–63. [17]
Stage 1 K_{max} < 48 D, thickness > 500 µm, absence of scarring.
Stage 2 K_{max} 48–53 D, thickness 400–500 µm, absence of scarring.
Stage 3 K_{max} 54–55 D, thickness 200–400 µm, absence of scarring.
Stage 4 $K_{max > 55}$ D, thickness < 200 µm, central corneal scarring.

Table 5.
Management algorithm in various stages of keratoconus.

5.2.3.3 Bowman layer transplantation

The PK or DALK may be disrupted by complications such as suture-related problems, graft rejection, epithelial wound-healing abnormalities, corneal curvature changes due to progression of KC in the peripheral host cornea resulting in disappointing visual results [86]. In KC corneas, pathological changes include the reduction of number of keratocytes, organization of the stromal lamellae, fragmentation or absent of Bowman's layer (BL) [91] It has been suggested that the BL may be the strongest biomechanical element of the human cornea followed by the anterior third of the cornea [92]. Therefore, the BL may play a structural role in maintaining the shape/tectonic stability in KC corneas [87]. This procedure was first described in 2014, Bowman's layer graft was positioned inside the recipient corneal stroma in a sandwich technique, without corneal incision or sutures, to pull the anterior corneal surface flatter and create homogeneous corneal topography [86]. BL transplantation can be performed under local anesthesia and low dose topical steroid can stop within 1 year post-operative, minimizing the risk of glaucoma development or cataract formation [86, 87, 93]. The reported complications are low such as intraoperative microperforation of the Descemet's membrane [87, 93]. Because of the transplanted tissue is acellular, no episodes of allograft rejection have been observed [86, 87]. This procedure may postpone penetrating keratoplasty (PK) or deep anterior lamellar keratoplasty (DALK) and potentially allowed long term contact lens wear [86]. Although graft preparation and surgical technique can be challenging, assisted technologies, such as femtosecond laser and intraoperative anterior segment optical coherence tomography (OCT), may help conquer these barriers [94, 95]. "Bowman layer onlay," a recently developed surgical technique in which an isolated Bowman's layer graft, is positioned onto the patient's anatomical Bowman's layer or anterior stroma, has demonstrated the rapid re-epithelization and integration of the tissue and comparable clinical outcomes to intrastromal transplantation [96]. The outcomes of each keratoplasty techniques are listed in **Table 4**.

There are a variety of nomograms for the treatment of keratoconus which are mainly focused on the keratoconus grading, risk factors, the progressive nature of the disease, and contact lens tolerance [15]. The management algorithm in various stages of keratoconus is shown in **Table 5**.

6. Future directions

Treatment for advanced KC has trended away from invasive procedures such as PK and even DALK toward minimally invasive procedures such as CXL, ICRS or BL transplantation. Although keratoconus is a multifactorial disease, the pathogenesis of the disease is very much affected by genetic factors and positive family history [2, 8, 97]. By identifying pathogenic genes and changing the structure of cell proteins, gene therapy may be a very promising and effective treatment modality to change the course of the disease [15].

7. Conclusion

The two most important goals of management of keratoconus are stopping disease progression and visual rehabilitation. An ocular allergy should be treated. Care providers should instruct the patients to avoid eye rubbing to halt disease progression. A careful follow up is needed to document disease progression and provide prompt treatment. A nonsurgical treatment of keratoconus includes spectacles or contact lens. Contact lens use does not slow or halt progression but can provide satisfactory vision in early stages of keratoconus. A contact lens type is selected based on the manifest refraction and the degree of keratoconus.

The five operations (CXL, ICRS, PK, DALK and BL transplantation) currently represent the available surgical treatment options for advanced KC. Treatment for advanced KC has trended away from invasive procedures such as PK and even DALK toward minimally invasive procedures such as CXL, ICRS or BL transplantation. CXL and ICRS were once regarded only for mild to moderate keratoconus, their roles are now expanding in advanced diseases as well.

PK and DALK provide long term good vision but has slow visual rehabilitation and may be disrupted by complications such as suture-related problems and graft rejection. BL transplantation was introduced for advanced KC with extreme thinning/steepening. This novel procedure may postpone penetrating keratoplasty (PK) or deep anterior lamellar keratoplasty (DALK) and potentially allow long term contact lens wear. Since genetic factors play significant roles in KC, advances in gene therapy may soon yield innovative treatments of this disease.

Author details

Vatookarn Roongpoovapatr[1,2]*, Mohamed Abou Shousha[2]
and Puwat Charukamnoetkanok[1]

1 Department of Ophthalmology, Mettapracharak (Wat Rai Khing) Hospital, Nakorn-Pathom, Thailand

2 Miller School of Medicine, Bascom Palmer Eye Institute, University of Miami, FL, USA

*Address all correspondence to: drvatookarn@gmail.com

References

[1] Rabinowitz YS. Keratoconus. Surv Ophthalmol. 1998;42:297-319.

[2] Davidson AE, Hayes S, Hardcastle AJ, Tuft SJ. The pathogenesis of keratoconus. Eye Lond Engl. 2014;28:189-95.

[3] Teng CC. Electron microscope study of the pathology of keratoconus: I. Am J Ophthalmol. 1963;55:18-47.

[4] Cozma I, Atherley C, James NJ. Influence of ethnic origin on the incidence of keratoconus and associated atopic disease in Asian and white patients. Eye Lond Engl. 2005;19:924-5; author reply 925-926.

[5] Georgiou T, Funnell CL, Cassels-Brown A, O'Conor R. Influence of ethnic origin on the incidence of keratoconus and associated atopic disease in Asians and white patients. Eye Lond Engl. 2004;18:379-83.

[6] Wang Y, Rabinowitz YS, Rotter JI, Yang H. Genetic epidemiological study of keratoconus: evidence for major gene determination. Am J Med Genet. 2000;93:403-9.

[7] Reinstein DZ, Archer TJ, Gobbe M. Corneal epithelial thickness profile in the diagnosis of keratoconus. J Refract Surg Thorofare NJ 1995. 2009;25:604-10.

[8] Ben-Eli H, Erdinest N, Solomon A. Pathogenesis and complications of chronic eye rubbing in ocular allergy: Curr Opin Allergy Clin Immunol. 2019;19:526-34.

[9] McMonnies CW. Mechanisms of rubbing-related corneal trauma in keratoconus. Cornea. 2009;28:607-15.

[10] Gomes JAP, Tan D, Rapuano CJ, Belin MW, Ambrósio R, Guell JL, et al. Global consensus on keratoconus and ectatic diseases. Cornea. 2015;34:359-69.

[11] Wang Y, Rabinowitz YS, Rotter JI, Yang H. Genetic epidemiological study of keratoconus: evidence for major gene determination. Am J Med Genet. 2000;93:403-9.

[12] Belin MW, Villavicencio OF, Ambrósio RR. Tomographic Parameters for the Detection of Keratoconus: Suggestions for Screening and Treatment Parameters. Eye Contact Lens Sci Clin Pract. 2014;40:326-30.

[13] Koc M, Tekin K, Tekin MI, Uzel MM, Kosekahya P, Ozulken K, et al. An Early Finding of Keratoconus: Increase in Corneal Densitometry. Cornea. 2018;37:580-6.

[14] Raiskup F, Theuring A, Pillunat LE, Spoerl E. Corneal collagen crosslinking with riboflavin and ultraviolet-A light in progressive keratoconus: ten-year results. J Cataract Refract Surg. 2015;41:41-6.

[15] Mohammadpour M, Heidari Z, Hashemi H. Updates on Managements for Keratoconus. J Curr Ophthalmol. 2018;30:110-24.

[16] Ishii R, Kamiya K, Igarashi A, Shimizu K, Utsumi Y, Kumanomido T. Correlation of corneal elevation with severity of keratoconus by means of anterior and posterior topographic analysis. Cornea. 2012;31:253-8.

[17] Krumeich JH, Daniel J, Knülle A. Live-epikeratophakia for keratoconus. J Cataract Refract Surg. 1998;24:456-63.

[18] Parker JS, van Dijk K, Melles GRJ. Treatment options for advanced keratoconus: A review. Surv Ophthalmol. 2015;60:459-80.

[19] Alió JL, Shabayek MH. Corneal higher order aberrations: a method to grade keratoconus. J Refract Surg Thorofare NJ 1995. 2006;22:539-45.

[20] McMahon TT, Szczotka-Flynn L, Barr JT, Anderson RJ, Slaughter ME, Lass JH, et al. A new method for grading the severity of keratoconus: the Keratoconus Severity Score (KSS). Cornea. 2006;25:794-800.

[21] Belin MW, Duncan JK. Keratoconus: The ABCD Grading System. Klin Monatsbl Augenheilkd. 2016;233:701-7.

[22] Martínez-Abad A, Piñero DP. New perspectives on the detection and progression of keratoconus. J Cataract Refract Surg. 2017;43:1213-27.

[23] Serrao S, Lombardo G, Calì C, Lombardo M. Role of corneal epithelial thickness mapping in the evaluation of keratoconus. Contact Lens Anterior Eye. 2019;42:662-5.

[24] Ozgurhan EB, Kara N, Yildirim A, Bozkurt E, Uslu H, Demirok A. Evaluation of corneal microstructure in keratoconus: a confocal microscopy study. Am J Ophthalmol. 2013;156:885-893.e2.

[25] Zhang X, Munir SZ, Sami Karim SA, Munir WM. A review of imaging modalities for detecting early keratoconus. Eye Lond Engl. 2020;

[26] El Rami H, Chelala E, Dirani A, Fadlallah A, Fakhoury H, Cherfan C, et al. An Update on the Safety and Efficacy of Corneal Collagen Cross-Linking in Pediatric Keratoconus. BioMed Res Int. 2015;2015:257927.

[27] Mastropasqua L. Collagen cross-linking: when and how? A review of the state of the art of the technique and new perspectives. Eye Vis Lond Engl. 2015;2:19.

[28] Maier P, Reinhard T, Kohlhaas M. Corneal Collagen Cross-Linking in the Stabilization of Keratoconus. Dtsch Arzteblatt Int. 2019;116:184-90.

[29] Pecorella I, Appolloni R, Tiezzi A, Plateroti P, Plateroti R. Histological Findings in a Failed Corneal Riboflavin–UVA Collagen Cross-linking Performed for Progressive Keratoconus: Cornea. 2013;32:191-5.

[30] Downie LE, Lindsay RG. Contact lens management of keratoconus. Clin Exp Optom. 2015;98:299-311.

[31] Rathi VM, Mandathara PS, Dumpati S. Contact lens in keratoconus. Indian J Ophthalmol. 2013;61:410-5.

[32] JN Buxton, DF Buxton, AK Dias. Keratoconus Basic and Clinical Features. The CLAO Guide to Basic Science and Clinical Practice.

[33] Perry HD, Buxton JN, Fine BS. Round and oval cones in keratoconus. Ophthalmology. 1980;87:905-9.

[34] B AlRomeih M. Piggyback Lens System in the Management of Keratoconus. Adv Ophthalmol Vis Syst [Internet]. 2015 [cited 2020 Sep 20];2. Available from: https://medcraveonline.com/AOVS/piggyback-lens-system-in-the-management-of-keratoconus.html

[35] Zhang X-H, Li X. Effect of rigid gas permeable contact lens on keratoconus progression: a review. Int J Ophthalmol. 2020;13:1124-31.

[36] Belin MW, Lim L, Rajpal RK, Hafezi F, Gomes JAP, Cochener B. Corneal Cross-Linking: Current USA Status: Report From the Cornea Society. Cornea. 2018;37:1218-25.

[37] Ziaei M, Barsam A, Shamie N, Vroman D, Kim T, Donnenfeld ED, et al. Reshaping procedures for the surgical management of corneal ectasia. J Cataract Refract Surg. 2015;41:842-72.

[38] Wollensak G, Spoerl E, Seiler T. Riboflavin/ultraviolet-a-induced collagen crosslinking for the treatment of keratoconus. Am J Ophthalmol. 2003;135:620-7.

[39] Subasinghe SK, Ogbuehi KC, Dias GJ. Current perspectives on corneal collagen crosslinking (CXL). Graefes Arch Clin Exp Ophthalmol Albrecht Von Graefes Arch Klin Exp Ophthalmol. 2018;256:1363-84.

[40] Sykakis E, Karim R, Evans JR, Bunce C, Amissah-Arthur KN, Patwary S, et al. Corneal collagen cross-linking for treating keratoconus. Cochrane Database Syst Rev. 2015;CD010621.

[41] Greenstein SA, Fry KL, Bhatt J, Hersh PS. Natural history of corneal haze after collagen crosslinking for keratoconus and corneal ectasia: Scheimpflug and biomicroscopic analysis. J Cataract Refract Surg. 2010;36:2105-14.

[42] Richoz O, Hammer A, Tabibian D, Gatzioufas Z, Hafezi F. The Biomechanical Effect of Corneal Collagen Cross-Linking (CXL) With Riboflavin and UV-A is Oxygen Dependent. Transl Vis Sci Technol. 2013;2:6.

[43] Shetty R, Pahuja NK, Nuijts RMMA, Ajani A, Jayadev C, Sharma C, et al. Current Protocols of Corneal Collagen Cross-Linking: Visual, Refractive, and Tomographic Outcomes. Am J Ophthalmol. 2015;160:243-9.

[44] Rubinfeld RS, Stulting RD, Gum GG, Talamo JH. Quantitative analysis of corneal stromal riboflavin concentration without epithelial removal. J Cataract Refract Surg. 2018;44:237-42.

[45] Davies E, Colby K. Controversies in Corneal Collagen Cross-linking. Int Ophthalmol Clin. 2015;55:1-11.

[46] Belviranli S, Oltulu R. Efficacy of pulsed-light accelerated crosslinking in the treatment of progressive keratoconus: Two-year results. Eur J Ophthalmol. 2019;1120672119872375.

[47] Al-Mohaimeed MM. Combined corneal CXL and photorefractive keratectomy for treatment of keratoconus: a review. Int J Ophthalmol. 2019;12:1929-38.

[48] Kobashi H, Rong SS. Corneal Collagen Cross-Linking for Keratoconus: Systematic Review. BioMed Res Int. 2017;2017:8145651.

[49] Meiri Z, Keren S, Rosenblatt A, Sarig T, Shenhav L, Varssano D. Efficacy of Corneal Collagen Cross-Linking for the Treatment of Keratoconus: A Systematic Review and Meta-Analysis. Cornea. 2016;35:417-28.

[50] Kanellopoulos AJ, Binder PS. Collagen cross-linking (CCL) with sequential topography-guided PRK: a temporizing alternative for keratoconus to penetrating keratoplasty. Cornea. 2007;26:891-5.

[51] Kanellopoulos AJ, Asimellis G. Epithelial remodeling after partial topography-guided normalization and high-fluence short-duration crosslinking (Athens protocol): results up to 1 year. J Cataract Refract Surg. 2014;40:1597-602.

[52] Kanellopoulos AJ. Comparison of sequential vs same-day simultaneous collagen cross-linking and topography-guided PRK for treatment of keratoconus. J Refract Surg Thorofare NJ 1995. 2009;25:S812-818.

[53] Singal N, Ong Tone S, Stein R, Bujak MC, Chan CC, Chew HF, et al. Comparison of accelerated CXL alone, accelerated CXL-ICRS, and accelerated CXL-TG-PRK in progressive keratoconus and other corneal ectasias. J Cataract Refract Surg. 2020;46:276-86.

[54] Henriquez MA, Izquierdo L, Bernilla C, McCarthy M. Corneal collagen cross-linking before Ferrara intrastromal corneal ring implantation for the treatment of

progressive keratoconus. Cornea. 2012;31:740-5.

[55] Hashemi H, Alvani A, SeyedianMA,YaseriM,KhabazkhoobM, Esfandiari H. Appropriate Sequence of Combined Intracorneal Ring Implantation and Corneal Collagen Cross-Linking in Keratoconus: A Systematic Review and Meta-Analysis. Cornea. 2018;37:1601-7.

[56] Assaf A, Kotb A. Simultaneous corneal crosslinking and surface ablation combined with phakic intraocular lens implantation for managing keratoconus. Int Ophthalmol. 2015;35:411-9.

[57] He C, Joergensen JS, Knorz MC, McKay KN, Zhang F. Three-Step Treatment of Keratoconus and Post-LASIK Ectasia: Implantation of ICRS, Corneal Cross-linking, and Implantation of Toric Posterior Chamber Phakic IOLs. J Refract Surg Thorofare NJ 1995. 2020;36:104-9.

[58] Abdelmassih Y, El-Khoury S, Chelala E, Slim E, Cherfan CG, Jarade E. Toric ICL Implantation After Sequential Intracorneal Ring Segments Implantation and Corneal Cross-linking in Keratoconus: 2-Year Follow-up. J Refract Surg Thorofare NJ 1995. 2017;33:610-6.

[59] Wollensak G. Crosslinking treatment of progressive keratoconus: new hope. Curr Opin Ophthalmol. 2006;17:356-60.

[60] Deshmukh R, Hafezi F, Kymionis GD, Kling S, Shah R, Padmanabhan P, et al. Current concepts in crosslinking thin corneas. Indian J Ophthalmol. 2019;67:8-15.

[61] Hafezi F, Mrochen M, Iseli HP, Seiler T. Collagen crosslinking with ultraviolet-A and hypoosmolar riboflavin solution in thin corneas. J Cataract Refract Surg. 2009;35:621-4.

[62] Li W, Wang B. Efficacy and safety of transepithelial corneal collagen crosslinking surgery versus standard corneal collagen crosslinking surgery for keratoconus: a meta-analysis of randomized controlled trials. BMC Ophthalmol. 2017;17:262.

[63] Buzzonetti L, Petrocelli G, Valente P, Iarossi G, Ardia R, Petroni S, et al. Iontophoretic Transepithelial Collagen Cross-Linking Versus Epithelium-Off Collagen Cross-Linking in Pediatric Patients: 3-Year Follow-Up. Cornea. 2019;38:859-63.

[64] Cagil N, Sarac O, Can GD, Akcay E, Can ME. Outcomes of corneal collagen crosslinking using a customized epithelial debridement technique in keratoconic eyes with thin corneas. Int Ophthalmol. 2017;37:103-9.

[65] Sachdev MS, Gupta D, Sachdev G, Sachdev R. Tailored stromal expansion with a refractive lenticule for crosslinking the ultrathin cornea. J Cataract Refract Surg. 2015;41:918-23.

[66] Jacob S, Kumar DA, Agarwal A, Basu S, Sinha P, Agarwal A. Contact lens-assisted collagen cross-linking (CACXL): A new technique for cross-linking thin corneas. J Refract Surg Thorofare NJ 1995. 2014;30:366-72.

[67] Lombardo M, Giannini D, Lombardo G, Serrao S. Randomized Controlled Trial Comparing Transepithelial Corneal Cross-linking Using Iontophoresis with the Dresden Protocol in Progressive Keratoconus. Ophthalmology. 2017;124:804-12.

[68] Sloot F, Soeters N, van der Valk R, Tahzib NG. Effective corneal collagen crosslinking in advanced cases of progressive keratoconus: J Cataract Refract Surg. 2013;39:1141-5.

[69] Soeters N, Wisse RPL, Godefrooij DA, Imhof SM, Tahzib NG. Transepithelial versus epithelium-off

corneal cross-linking for the treatment of progressive keratoconus: a randomized controlled trial. Am J Ophthalmol. 2015;159:821-828.e3.

[70] Arora R, Jain P, Goyal JL, Gupta D. Comparative Analysis of Refractive and Topographic Changes in Early and Advanced Keratoconic Eyes Undergoing Corneal Collagen Crosslinking. Cornea. 2013;32:1359-64.

[71] Piñero DP, Alio JL, Klonowski P, Toffaha B. Vectorial astigmatic changes after corneal collagen crosslinking in keratoconic corneas previously treated with intracorneal ring segments: a preliminary study. Eur J Ophthalmol. 2012;22 Suppl 7:S69-80.

[72] Toprak I, Yildirim C. Effects of corneal collagen crosslinking on corneal topographic indices in patients with keratoconus. Eye Contact Lens. 2013;39:385-7.

[73] Al Fayez MF, Alfayez S, Alfayez Y. Transepithelial Versus Epithelium-Off Corneal Collagen Cross-Linking for Progressive Keratoconus: A Prospective Randomized Controlled Trial. Cornea. 2015;34 Suppl 10:S53-56.

[74] Craig JA, Mahon J, Yellowlees A, Barata T, Glanville J, Arber M, et al. Epithelium-off photochemical corneal collagen cross-linkage using riboflavin and ultraviolet a for keratoconus and keratectasia: a systematic review and meta-analysis. Ocul Surf. 2014;12:202-14.

[75] Yuksel E, Cubuk MO, Yalcin NG. Accelerated epithelium-on or accelerated epithelium-off corneal collagen cross-linking: Contralateral comparison study. Taiwan J Ophthalmol. 2020;10:37-44.

[76] Nicula CA, Nicula D, Rednik AM, Bulboacă AE. Comparative Results of "Epi-Off" Conventional versus "Epi-Off" Accelerated Cross-Linking Procedure at 5-year Follow-Up. J Ophthalmol. 2020;2020:4745101.

[77] Bowes O, Coutts S, Ismailjee A, Trocme E, Vilella AJ, Perry H, et al. Pulsed Light Accelerated Corneal Collagen Cross-Linking: 1-Year Results. Cornea. 2017;36:e15-6.

[78] Jiang Y, Yang S, Li Y, Cui G, Lu TC. Accelerated Versus Conventional Corneal Collagen Cross-Linking in the Treatment of Keratoconus: A Meta-analysis and Review of the Literature. Interdiscip Sci Comput Life Sci. 2019;11:282-6.

[79] Shajari M, Kolb CM, Agha B, Steinwender G, Müller M, Herrmann E, et al. Comparison of standard and accelerated corneal cross-linking for the treatment of keratoconus: a meta-analysis. Acta Ophthalmol (Copenh). 2019;97:e22-35.

[80] Torquetti L, Ferrara G, Almeida F, Cunha L, Araujo LPN, Machado AP, et al. Intrastromal corneal ring segments implantation in patients with keratoconus: 10-year follow-up. J Refract Surg Thorofare NJ 1995. 2014;30:22-6.

[81] Liu H, Chen Y, Wang P, Li B, Wang W, Su Y, et al. Efficacy and safety of deep anterior lamellar keratoplasty vs. penetrating keratoplasty for keratoconus: a meta-analysis. PloS One. 2015;10:e0113332.

[82] Tuft SJ, Gregory W. Long-term refraction and keratometry after penetrating keratoplasty for keratoconus. Cornea. 1995;14:614-7.

[83] Bedi R, Touboul D, Pinsard L, Colin J. Refractive and topographic stability of Intacs in eyes with progressive keratoconus: five-year follow-up. J Refract Surg Thorofare NJ 1995. 2012;28:392-6.

[84] Fukuoka S, Honda N, Ono K, Mimura T, Usui T, Amano S. Extended

long-term results of penetrating keratoplasty for keratoconus. Cornea. 2010;29:528-30.

[85] Niziol LM, Musch DC, Gillespie BW, Marcotte LM, Sugar A. Long-term outcomes in patients who received a corneal graft for keratoconus between 1980 and 1986. Am J Ophthalmol. 2013;155:213-219.e3.

[86] van Dijk K, Parker J, Tong CM, Ham L, Lie JT, Groeneveld-van Beek EA, et al. Midstromal isolated Bowman layer graft for reduction of advanced keratoconus: a technique to postpone penetrating or deep anterior lamellar keratoplasty. JAMA Ophthalmol. 2014;132:495-501.

[87] van Dijk K, Liarakos VS, Parker J, Ham L, Lie JT, Groeneveld-van Beek EA, et al. Bowman Layer Transplantation to Reduce and Stabilize Progressive, Advanced Keratoconus. Ophthalmology. 2015;122:909-17.

[88] Hashemi H, Jabbarvand M, Kheirkhah A, Yazdani-Abyaneh A, Beheshtnejad A, Ghaffary S. Efficacy of intacs intrastromal corneal ring segment relative to depth of insertion evaluated with anterior segment optical coherence tomography. Middle East Afr J Ophthalmol. 2013;20:234.

[89] Jacob S, Patel SR, Agarwal A, Ramalingam A, Saijimol AI, Raj JM. Corneal Allogenic Intrastromal Ring Segments (CAIRS) Combined With Corneal Cross-linking for Keratoconus. J Refract Surg Thorofare NJ 1995. 2018;34:296-303.

[90] Henein C, Nanavaty MA. Systematic review comparing penetrating keratoplasty and deep anterior lamellar keratoplasty for management of keratoconus. Contact Lens Anterior Eye J Br Contact Lens Assoc. 2017;40:3-14.

[91] Sherwin T, Brookes NH. Morphological changes in keratoconus: pathology or pathogenesis. Clin Experiment Ophthalmol. 2004;32:211-7.

[92] Marshall J. The 2014 Bowman Lecture-Bowman's and Bruch's: a tale of two membranes during the laser revolution. Eye Lond Engl. 2015;29:46-64.

[93] Dragnea DC, Birbal RS, Ham L, Dapena I, Oellerich S, van Dijk K, et al. Bowman layer transplantation in the treatment of keratoconus. Eye Vis Lond Engl. 2018;5:24.

[94] Dapena I, Parker JS, Melles GRJ. Potential benefits of modified corneal tissue grafts for keratoconus: Bowman layer "inlay" and "onlay" transplantation, and allogenic tissue ring segments. Curr Opin Ophthalmol. 2020;31:276-83.

[95] García de Oteyza G, González Dibildox LA, Vázquez-Romo KA, Tapia Vázquez A, Dávila Alquisiras JH, Martínez-Báez BE, et al. Bowman layer transplantation using a femtosecond laser. J Cataract Refract Surg. 2019;45:261-6.

[96] Tong CM, van Dijk K, Melles GRJ. Update on Bowman layer transplantation. Curr Opin Ophthalmol. 2019;30:249-55.

[97] Ferrari G, Rama P. The keratoconus enigma: A review with emphasis on pathogenesis. Ocul Surf. 2020;18:363-73.

Chapter 4

Advances in Non-surgical Treatment Methods in Vision Rehabilitation of Keratoconus Patients

Ersin Muhafiz

Abstract

Visual acuity decreases due to progressive irregular astigmatism in keratoconus (KC). Although glasses can be useful in the initial stages of vision rehabilitation, contact lenses (CL) are needed in many patients due to irregular astigmatism. Although rigid gas permeable (RGP) CLs provided the patient with a better visual acuity than glasses, their effects on corneal tissues and caused comfort problems. Although soft CL produced for KC have solved some of these problems, they could not increase visual acuity as much as RGPs in advanced stage KC. For this reason, new searches for vision rehabilitation and comfort in KC have continued. In this context, piggyback contact lenses (PBCL) have been used in vision rehabilitation. Hybrid CLs have gained popularity due to the fact that PBCLs cause corneal neovascularization and giant papillary conjunctivitis. Scleral CLs have been developed for limited benefit in some patients with advanced KC. Scleral CLs provided good vision rehabilitation. The biggest problem of scleral CLs is the application and removal difficulty. All these CL modalities try to improve the quality of life and delay surgical procedures by increasing the level of vision in patients with KC.

Keywords: spectacles, rigid gas permeable contact lens, soft contact lens, hybrid contact lens, scleral contact lens, piggyback contact lens

1. Introduction

Keratoconus (KC) is the most common ectatic disease of the cornea. It is characterized by progressive thinning and protrusion of the cornea [1, 2]. Consequently, irregular astigmatism, myopia and a decrease in visual acuity occur. Therefore, the disease has a negative effect on vision-related quality of life. The disease has become an important public health problem due to the economic burden of treatment and vision rehabilitation related processes [3]. KC in children may have negative effects on social and educational development. In this respect, it is necessary to improve the vision in children at an acceptable level [4].

This disease, which mostly starts in young adults, can also be seen in children. It stabilizes in the fourth-fifth decades of life. KC, which usually shows bilateral asymmetric involvement, can be asymptomatic at the beginning, and visual acuity decreases as the disease progresses [1, 2]. Although some systemic involvement of

KC is shown, it is generally known as a local corneal disease [5, 6]. Abnormalities in the corneal epithelium, Bowman's layer and especially the collagen structure of the stroma play a role in the pathogenesis of the disease. Although it is suggested that various biochemical and genetic factors play a role in the etiology, its exact cause is not known exactly. The main diagnostic method of KC is placido disc-based corneal topography [2, 5, 7].

While surgical options in KC management aim to change the natural course of the disease and increase vision, the main goal of non-surgical options is to improve vision without damaging the ocular surface. Classical non-surgical treatment of vision rehabilitation in KC is glasses in a small number of patients and CLs in the majority of patients. In addition, modern surgical options such as intraocular lens implantation, corneal cross-linking (CXL), intra-stromal rings and anterior lamellar keratoplasty are also used in treatment. The common feature of these surgical methods is that they increase visual rehabilitation to a certain level due to residual refraction after surgery and ongoing irregular astigmatism, even if they are performed very successfully. Therefore, CLs are needed for vision rehabilitation after surgical methods [2, 7, 8].

Today, there is a global consensus that CLs play the most important role in the visual rehabilitation of KC patients [8]. Later developments in CL design and materials expanded the application options for KC patients. Considering that CLs cause ocular surface changes even in non-KC individuals, the main purpose of CL application in KC should be to increase visual acuity without compromising the health of the cornea and ocular surface [9]. While the patient should have good vision and comfort with the lens, the practitioner must find a suitable lens fitting that does not compromise the anterior ocular surface health. Therefore, the process is often time-consuming and difficult for both the patient and the ophthalmologist. Due to the nature of long-term CL use in KC, a careful CL selection should be made considering the physiological needs of the cornea according to the level of ectasia. Since CL movements can cause mechanical effects on the cornea with CL movements during millions of blinking, it is necessary to ensure that CL applies minimal contact and pressure on the cone in KC patients. In addition, since there are stem cells in the limbus region, which are hallmarks of corneal physiology and regeneration, contact with the limbal region should be minimized in order to prevent CLs from damaging the limbal region [2]. Scheimpflug imaging and anterior segment optical coherence tomography, which are frequently used in ophthalmology practice in recent years, can be used to evaluate CL fit. These imaging technologies can be used to reduce the time we spend evaluating CL fitting and to improve guides for CL fitting [10].

In addition to the severity of the KC, it is decided which type of CL will be selected according to the visual demand and comfort of the patient and the CL tolerance. With the latest advances in CL features and design, many CL options have been developed for patients with corneal irregularities, such as large diameter RGP lenses, scleral lenses, hybrid lenses and KC specific soft lenses. New data reveal that special design CLs, new design scleral lenses and hybrid lenses provide better visual acuity as well as better comfort than traditional RGPs [2, 8, 11].

2. Advances in non-surgical treatment methods in vision rehabilitation of keratoconus patients

2.1 Spectacles

Since astigmatism is mild in the early stages of KC, vision can be corrected with glasses. However, as irregular astigmatism increases in the middle and advanced stages, vision decreases dramatically and glasses play a limited role in correcting vision. In addition, since the disease is usually asymmetrical, correction with glasses can lead to anisometropia and anzioconia. Therefore, it is necessary to evaluate CL options for a better vision [8, 11, 12]. Glasses can only be given to selected patients who are intolerant to CL and who are not willing to undergo any surgery. Glasses can be prescribed on soft CL in some KC patients. Depending on the developments in CL technologies, the decrease in side effects due to CL and the effect of increased comfort may cause patients in the initial KC stage who can benefit from glasses nowadays to turn to CL. Because we can observe that CLs are frequently preferred instead of glasses due to esthetic concerns [11–13]. However it has been suggested that wearing rigid gas permeable CL (RGP) will increase the irregularities in the cornea and cloud the central cornea due to low corneal stiffness in KC patients under the age of 20. In order to prevent these problems, it has been stated that when visual impairment is detected in KC patients under the age of 20, it should be corrected with glasses as much as possible [14].

2.2 Soft contact lenses

Conventional spherical or toric soft contact lenses (SCL) can provide benefit in improving vision by correcting myopia and regular astigmatism in early stage or form-frusted KC. Since they transfer the irregularities in the anterior surface of the cornea to their anterior surfaces, their ability to correct irregular astigmatism, high-order aberrations and vision level is very low in the KC, and therefore it limits the use of conventional SCLs in the KC. These conventional SCLs are generally ideal for those with a visual acuity of 1.0 with glasses [2]. They may be beneficial in some situations where high myopia is associated with KC disease [13]. After CXL treatment, they can assist in early vision rehabilitation. Hydrogel SCLs can be used in situations where comfort is more important [2]. The success of these lenses can be checked with a topography to be made over the lens. Depending on the needs of the patient, hydrogels with high water content and silicone hydrogel lenses with high oxygen permeability can be selected.

Developments in production technologies and specific basic curve designs have enabled the development of SCL specific to KC [15]. New design SCLs, customized hydrogel SCLs and pin-hole SCLs have expanded the usage spectrum of SCLs in KC [11]. It has also been found that they have similar quality of life between RGPs and SCLs [16]. Because of their good centralization, they can be used in decentralized cones and large diameter cones. In KC, it helps to increase visual acuity by making the anterior optic surface (front lens surface) more homogeneous topographically and by reducing high-order aberrations. In some sophisticated SCLs (customized SCL), asymmetric optical correction is performed, aberrations are further reduced and a better vision is achieved [17]. These special SCLs designed for KC have a greater central thickness than conventional SCLs (between 0.3 mm and 0.6 mm). This central thickness helps the CL to have a more stable structure and a regular anterior surface is tried to be created by preventing the direct adaptation of the lens on the irregular cornea. Increasing CL thickness contributes to the increase of visual performance, but also causes a decrease in oxygen permeability. This increases the risk of developing possible complications due to hypoxia. Therefore, they have a thinner peripheral thickness that can be adjusted independently of the silicone hydrogel central part and provides comfort with the movement of the lens. Since they are designed for use in KC, options with high spherical and toric values are available [12]. HydroCone® (Toris K) (SwissLens, Prilly, Switzerland) and KeraSoft® IC (Bausch & Lomb Inc., Rochester, NY) are silicone hydrogel SCLs specially designed for KC [18, 19]. It has been reported that with these lenses, visual acuity at a similar degree to RGPs is obtained in KC [15, 19]. It has been shown that SCLs increase vision in a significant portion of patients with corneal ring implantation. In cases where satisfactory vision cannot be achieved with SCLs, PBCL systems can be used in these patients [20].

It has been reported that visual performance decreases when the movement of the SCL exceeds 0.5 mm after blinking. Therefore, the movement of these lenses is requested not to exceed 0.5 mm, which may limit the tear change under the lens [12, 21]. These lenses, in which a sufficient visual level is obtained, have low infection rates due to a sufficient tear exchange. Although they provide more comfort, low oxygen permeability (excluding silicone hydrogels) compared to RGPs, failure to correct severe irregular astigmatism is the biggest disadvantage of SCLs [12]. As a result, with the developments in recent years, comfortable use and high visual performance have been achieved with SCLs specially produced for KC. However, it seems that the use of SCLs in KC will increase with future developments.

2.3 Rigid gas permeable contact lenses

RGPs are the most frequently used CLs in the world to increase the vision level in KC. In a study, it was found that RGPs delay surgical interventions in 98.9% of KC patients [8, 22]. Today, there are various RGPs developed for KC, including multicurve, asferic and quadrant-specific designs [23]. The lens has a steeper central curvature, a flatter peripheral curve, and they have a non-fused surface appearance. It is indicated in KC patients in whom glasses or SCLs fail to improve vision [24]. RGPs provide a better vision in KC patients compared to glasses [25]. It has also been reported that it controls the progression of the disease with its mild shaping effect [22, 26]. Providing a smooth spherical anterior optic surface, RGP helps maintain the shape of the cornea by applying light pressure to the cone area (**Figure 1**). In addition, optically low order astigmatism and high order aberrations are corrected with the tear fluid under the lens. Thus, contrast sensitivity and visual acuity increases. When the limbal region is desired to be protected, corneal RGPs are placed in most cases because they do not have any interaction with the limbal region [12, 27, 28].

The tear film under the lens is observed with fluorescent dye and the fitting can be evaluated and easily applied by an experienced practitioner. The disadvantage of these lenses is that the contrast sensitivity is low due to high-order aberrations, even if the visual acuity is good when the centralization is not good or when there is a tilt. To overcome this, RGPs with large optical zone (7.50–8.00) have been produced. Moreover, lenses with aspherical surfaces that correspond to the ectatic cornea have been produced with increased diameter up to 10.00–11.00 mm. Large diameter lenses are more complex to fit. Better fittings are obtained with small central or

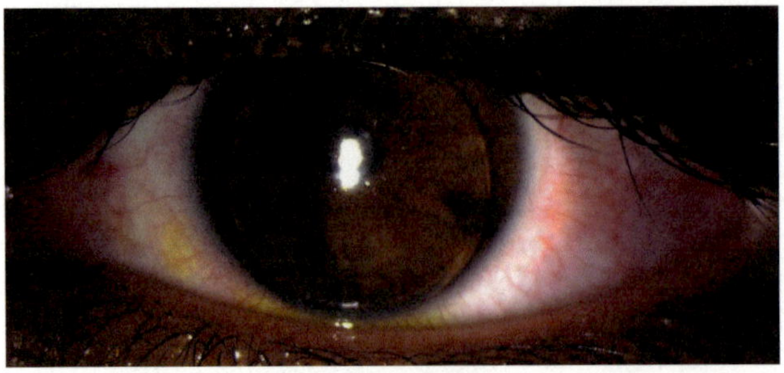

Figure 1.
Rigid gas permeable contact lens on the cornea providing a smooth anterior optic surface.

light cones [16, 29]. Dynamic and static fit should be evaluated 30 minutes after the CL is inserted. In dynamic fit, the centralization of the lens, its movement by blinking, and its stability in gaze positions are evaluated. The movement of the lens should not be more than 1 mm, it should not pass the limbus and its comfort should be maintained. In static fit, fluorescein is used to evaluate apical clearance, apical bearing, or three point touch [13]. Corneal astigmatism and higher order aberrations are reduced in all three methods. A larger diameter and flatter base curve is selected for apical bearing. The lens is directly supported by the corneal apex, and epithelial damage to the cornea secondary to the harsh between the lens and the corneal apex may develop an apical scar [30]. In this method, which provides a better visual quality, there is a risk of apical scarring. In apical clearance, a lens with a steeper base curve and smaller diameter is selected from the cornea, and the lens is supported by the cornea paracentral and there is a clear area between the central cornea and the lens. In this application where the risk of central corneal scar formation is reduced, tightening at periphery cornea may restrict tear exchange and may lead to hypoxic complications. In the three point touch method, which is the most popular method, the lens is supported mostly by the peripheral cornea and very little by the corneal apex [23, 31, 32]. In this method, attention should be paid to prevent contact of the lens with the corneal apex. Monocurve RGPs are used in mild to medium KC, and multicurve CLs are used in advanced KC. However, in some advanced KC, fitting of corneal RGPs may be more difficult and lens decentralization, dislocation, and disconfort may be encountered [33].

They can lead to a corneal warpage, especially in long-term use [34]. It can be a little difficult to get optimum comfort as it is made of rigid material only. There are studies showing that there is no relationship between KC severity and patient comfort, as well as studies showing that the opposite is valid [35–37]. Special cone-designed lenses such as Rose-K enabled RGPs to be very effective in visual acuity [38]. It has been reported that RGPs aggravate dry eye signs and symptoms in KC patients [39]. Since we may encounter a completely new eye after keratoplasty in liver patients, graft characteristics may make corneal RGPs contraindicated [40]. PBCL systems or scleral CLs can be used in these situations. RGPs allow for a good tear exchange. In advanced cases, a better vision can be obtained than SCLs, but discomfort, foreign body sensation and poor fitting in some advanced cases, especially in decentralized cones, are disadvantages of difficulty in centralization. Despite this, RGPs continue to be the first-line treatment in the visual rehabilitation of KC patients [8].

2.4 Piggyback contact lenses

Piggyback contact lenses (PBCL) contain two CLs in one eye, one soft CL on the cornea and RGP above the soft CL. Thus, the optical performance of RGP and the comfort of SCL are utilized. It is thought that the placement of an SCL under the RGP protects the cornea from the excessive pressure of the RGP, thus minimizing this possible complication of RGP use and increasing comfort. If the patient has residual astigmatism, residual astigmatism can be placed in the SCL (toric) in the PBCL system and thus a spherical RGP can be used. It has also been suggested that the use of SCL with high positive power will help improve the centralization of RGP on the keratoconic cornea especially in KC patients with inferior cone [13, 23]. PBCLs can be used as an alternative option in patients with intolerance to RGPs due to ocular surface disorders, and eyes that cannot be stabilized with RGP and staining at 3–9 o'clock. It is also indicated in keratoplasty and KC patients in whom rehabilitation cannot be achieved with RGP [13]. It has been detected that 2% of KC patients using CL used PBCL [13, 41]. They may also help increase vision in KC patients with a corneal ring [42]. First, a soft CL (preferably a silicone hydrogel with minus power) is inserted, in which optimum fitting is achieved. This SCL covers the entire cornea, providing a bandage effect that helps protect the KC apex and a better centralization. Therefore, PBCL systems provide better comfort and longer duration of use, although their visual acuity is similar compared to RGP alone [12]. The base curve of the RGP is selected according to the values in the topography and keratometry applied over this soft CL, and it is inserted over this soft CL. After the RGP is inserted, the compatibility of the lenses with each other is evaluated using fluorescein dye. By changing the power of the soft CL, the compatibility of the RGP can be changed. For example, a positive powered soft CL can be used to flatten the RGP, and a negative powered RGP can be used to steep the base curve of RGP [13, 43]. Most practitioners use a low positive power SCL as it is considered to facilitate the centralization of RGP. However, it has also been suggested that the use of negative powered SCLs in the PBCL system results in better oxygen transmission. Refraction is measured over the two lenses and subjective refraction providing the best visual acuity is added to the RGP power [44, 45]. For an optimal fitting, it needs to move independently but harmoniously with blinking at the slit lamp and have minimal touch in the pattern of fluorescence. This independent movement allows tear exchange between the lenses, allowing the use of dissolved oxygen in the tear [46, 47]. In order to reduce the risk of hypoxia, care should be taken to ensure that both lenses have a high Dk value. In addition, there are custom PBCLs produced by opening a groove where RGP will sit on the soft CL to increase the centralization of RGP. Since the edges of the RGP fit into the groove in these lenses, they can provide better comfort [13]. PBCL improves vision and comfort, but potential hypoxia-related problems are among its disadvantages due to the application of maintenance procedures for both lenses and the double barrier that prevents oxygen transmission to the cornea. Today, a combination of high DK silicone hydrogel SLC and high Dk RGP is often preferred to prevent hypoxia complications [47, 48]. Although the corneal epithelium and endothelium are not affected in this system, giant papillary conjunctivitis and corneal neovascularization may develop in some patients due to the presence of two lenses on the corneal surface [2].

2.5 Hybrid contact lenses

Hybrid contact lenses (HCL) consist of a combination of a rigid central zone and a soft peripheral skirt, manufactured using special technology. In these lenses, it tries to benefit from the best features of RGP (better vision) and soft materials (comfort). Therefore, HCLs can be an effective alternative to RGP and PBCLs. There are many special applications and designs that provide successful results in irregular corneas such as KC with these lenses [12, 49]. Modern HCLs are indicated when there is RGP intolerance or poor centralization, when an optimal RGP fit cannot be achieved, when there is reduced daily wearing time of RGP. They have also been shown to help improve vision after keratoplasty [33, 50]. Since these lenses with central RGP function and have soft peripheral skirt, they provide comfort as well as correcting vision. Therefore, they are preferred by many physicians and patients. Due to their design, HCLs distribute the contact equally between the cornea and conjunctiva or only touch the conjunctiva and peripheral cornea. Hybrid lenses generally consist of an 8.00 mm rigid part in the center and a soft hydrogel part with a total diameter of 14.50 mm. Correction principles are similar to those of RGPs. A good centralization is achieved in hybrid lenses owing to their soft skirt. However, they require special training and practice for successful application [2, 49, 50].

SynergEyes® Ultrahealth (SynergEyes Inc., Carlsbad, CA) HCLs are the next generation hybrid CLs that have been developed with a base curve design (KC), stronger RGP/silicone hydrogel coupling, and higher Dk of the central and peripheral region. Thus, hypoxia and fusion line tears are prevented. In the KC, the Vault of the rigid component and the skirt curvature of the soft component can be adjusted separately. In these lenses with a vault value ranging from 100 to 600 microns, optimum fitting is achieved with a full apical clearance with fluorescein dye and without air bubbles under the lens and a soft landing in the fusion area [12, 23]. There should be no air bubbles in the middle of the lens and a light touch on the rigid-soft junction. Unlike RGP lenses, the hybrid systems centralize the optics regardless of the cone position. Therefore it can be used in most central and decentralized cones. In this design, a steeper skirt enhances lens movement and prevents it from sticking. The data obtained from the corneal topography can be used to estimate the parameters when placing these lenses.

It has been shown in some studies that HCLs, which have the most superior features of comfort compared to RGPs, provide better visual acuity and contrast sensitivity than RGPs. For this reason, it has been stated that they have a higher vision-related quality of life score than RGPs. Disadvantages include giant papillary conjunctivitis and tearing of the soft skirt, corneal clouding [11, 51, 52]. In summary, HCLs serve the purpose of combining the superior features of rigid and soft CLs in a single lens. However, since studies in this area are limited, further research is needed.

2.6 Scleral contact lenses

The diameters of full scleral lenses range from 18.1–25.0 mm and have a scleral bed and maximum corneal clearance. Miniscleral lenses have scleral bed and minimal corneal clearance, with diameters between 15.0–18.0 mm. Semiscleral lenses have scleral and corneal beds and their diameters are between 13.6 and 14.9 mm. The corneoscleral lenses touch the corneal bed and sclera with a diameter between 12.9 and 13.5 mm [43]. Existing scleral lenses are produced from materials with high oxygen permeability such as fluorosilicon acrylate [53]. As the thickness of the lens increases, the oxygen permeability decreases, so nowadays it has become possible to make thin lens designs with new software. In addition, the lens surface is coated with plasma, increasing the surface wettability, thus increasing comfort and daily wearing time. Today, they can be produced with a very smoother surface and edge structure and less deficits during construction. Technological developments in lens materials, designs and lens production, lens placement techniques have led to an increase in interest in these lenses and increased acceptability of lenses in the treatment of KC [54, 55].

Scleral lenses rest on the sclera, do not touch the cornea and limbus, and leave a clear space between the cornea and the lens. Before the lens is placed in the eye, it is filled with a preservative-free saline. The lens consists of three parts: the optical part, the part extending over the sclera (haptic) and the Vault responsible for the corneal and limbal clearance of the lens. The optical part of the scleral contact lens (S-CL) is generally desired to be 0.2 mm larger than the horizontal visible iris diameter. However, it is also of great importance that the haptic part, which is more important in the fitting, and the corneal and limbal vault are appropriate for stabilization of vision [54, 55]. Today, the most commonly used S-CL fitting method is performed by the use of fitting trial sets. In addition, lens manufacturers can recommend a suitable guide. S-CLs mask irregular anterior corneal surface astigmatism with the fluid reservoir. The most important issue in applying these lenses is their alignment to the sclera. In some patients, edge lifts due to the toric structure of the sclera can be observed. Today, S-CLs with quadrant-specific peripheral designs can be produced for these KC patients with scleral asymmetry. This increases the comfort and lens wearing time of patients [56]. With the advances in CLs, S-CLs are also available today for elderly KC patients to rehabilitate near vision [8, 57]. However, studies on these are limited. Production of these specially designed lenses is still quite difficult, as they require special equipment and training and high cost [54].

Since the S-CL fits on the bulbar conjunctiva, minimal tear change occurs under the lens. The generally accepted minimum diameter for the cornea and limbal area to be unpressurized is 16 mm. Optical correction in these lenses is provided by the liquid under the well centralized lens. Therefore, anterior optical aberrations of the keratoconic cornea are neutralized. Front surface eccentricity in S-CLs aims to correct the optical quality and vision by compensating the back surface anomalies in the KC. Front surface eccentricity is zero in a spherical lens. Higher front surface eccentricity values indicate that the lens flattens rapidly from the center to the periphery [2, 27, 54, 58]. Providing continuous lubrication of the whole corneal surface ensures the stabilization of visual acuity [59]. S-CLs eliminate high grade aberrations and provide good centering and improve the visual quality. The complexity of the usage procedures and the poor comfort in long-term use limit their use [54]. S-CLs are generally not the first CLs to be applied in KC. They are preferred when tolerance problems are experienced with other CLs (SCL, RGP, PBCLs) or when acceptable vision cannot be obtained [49, 53, 54, 59]. S-CLs are indicated in RGP intolerance, very advanced and decentered cones, cornea staining at 3–9 o'clock, vascularization with PBCL, advanced KC. The fact that it is indicated in the presence of ocular surface disorder and in severe dry eye further expands the areas of use in the KC [60]. Corneal vaulting, centralization and perfect comfort have led to the preference of S-CLs in less severe cases, thus widening the indication for use of S-CLs in KC. S-CL designs are generally preferred after all corneal surgeries in the liver (CXL, intracorneal ring, keratoplasty). In such cases, higher Vault may be preferred if the ring or graft junction or sutures are to be protected [61–63]. If success is not achieved with these lenses, surgical methods are used. Contraindications are corneal edema due to decreased endothelial count, hydrops, and previous filtration surgery. Scleral lenses show success in extremely irregular and steep corneas because of their large diameters. Therefore, the role of treatment is increasing in advanced ectatic corneas where there is no option other than surgery. In addition, due to their large diameter and vaults, they are more comfortable than RGPs since they do not directly contact the cornea, which has much more innervation than the sclera. In recent years, new S-CL designs have expanded the scope of CL use in KC patients [11, 13].

Miniscleral lenses have less corneal opening than full scleral lenses. Small diameter lenses tend to adhere to the cornea due to the suction vacuum, which may cause difficulties for the practitioner [54, 64]. It has been shown that S-CLs reduce the need for keratoplasty and patients are successfully treated with S-CL instead of keratoplasty [65]. When the effect of CL on quality of life was evaluated in liver patients, it was seen that RGP, hybrid, soft CL had a similar effect. S-CLs are more comfortable than these lenses, but midday fogging continues to limit the quality of life in these lenses. In addition, unlike these lenses, S-CLs have been reported to reduce dry eye signs and symptoms [60, 66].

Haptic and vault are evaluated under biomicroscope in S-CLs. An acceptable fitting is defined by a corneal clearance, no air bubbles underneath, and no compression of the conjunctiva veins. After obtaining the appropriate fit, a trial use of 4–6 hours is required to evaluate the KC patient's comfort and visual quality. A 400–600 micron Vault is acceptable for scleral lenses. However, a slightly higher vault may be prescribed due to the detection of a decrease in the vault after four hours of use and also considering that KC may progress over time. A convenient central and peripheral vault ensures patient comfort and tolerability. Feeling suction while removing the lens after four hours of CL application and the presence of staining in the conjunctiva are indicators of choosing a flatter haptic. It is recommended that patients be examined again 3–4 weeks after removing the lens to make a final decision [13].

Disadvantages are maintenance procedures, frequent replacement of saline bottles, insertion regimes using plungers, which can be more cumbersome than other methods, reduced tear exchange, and high costs. S-CLs in KC can cause infectious keratitis or other adverse events. It has been suggested that this may be due to inadequate cleaning of the plunger used for inserting and removing the lens and improper use of saline solution [8, 67, 68].

3. The role of new imaging technologies in contact lens fitting in keratoconus

First of all, the data on the radii of curvature obtained in the corneal topography can be helpful in determining the initial base curve when placing the RGP. By evaluating the size and localization of the cone in the KC with the help of tangential maps in the topography, a more appropriate RGP diameter and base curve can be selected [69]. It has been reported that these data in the topography are also useful in hybrid lens fitting in KC [70]. These systems also include CL fitting simulation software to model the possible effects of lens designs and changes in parameters on the fitting. Rigid lens fluorescein simulations are based on corneal elevation data modeled on tangential maps. There are also studies showing that the video keratoscopic system gives successful results from standard methods in RGP fitting when compared to standard procedures. It was determined that the virtual sodium fluorescein staining pattern created based on the data from the CL simulator in the corneal topography and the actual staining pattern observed in the slit lamp were found to be highly matched. These findings show the importance of video keratoscopic virtual applications in CL management in KC patients and they have the potential to reduce the time we spend for CL [23, 71].

Previously, corneal clearance could roughly be estimated by comparing it with the thickness of the cornea. Today, with new technological devices such as anterior segment optical coherence tomography (AS-OCT), the amount of corneal clearance can be measured much more accurately (**Figure 2**). It is stated that the vault changed over time after the S-CL was inserted. It is important to follow this with

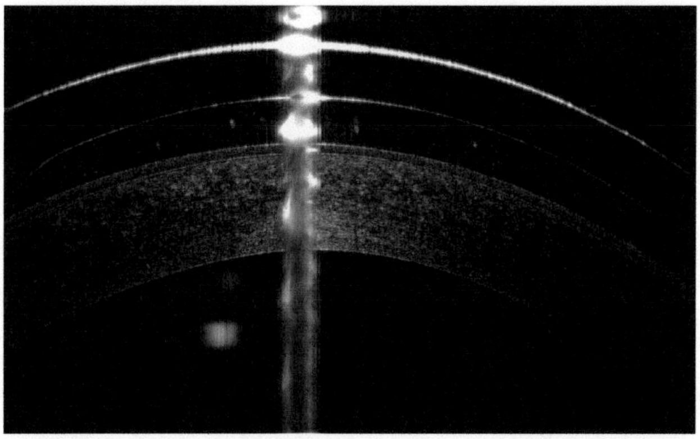

Figure 2.
Anterior segment-optical coherence tomography image showing corneal clearance in a hybrid contact lens wearer.

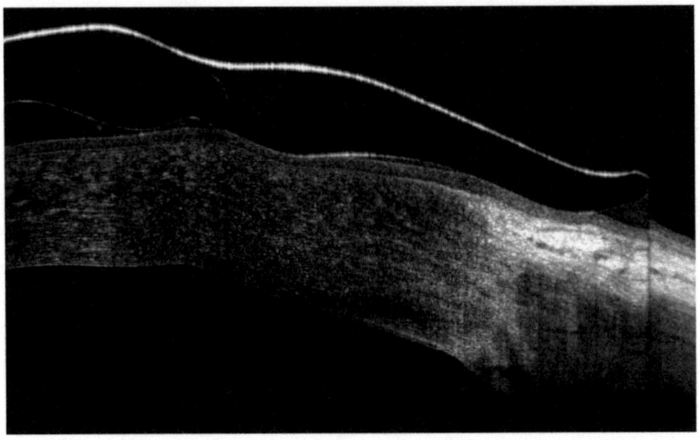

Figure 3.
Anterior segment-optical coherence tomography image showing the interaction between the contact lens corneal and the conjunctival surface in a hybrid contact lens wearer.

AS-OCT in progressive diseases such as KC. Because, in patients with KC, with the advancement of the cone and the decrease of the Vault, it may cause the touch between the cornea and the lens, corneal scarring and decreased vision. Therefore, the idea (owing to AS-OCT) that lenses can be used for a long time by increasing the vault has emerged in KC patients [54, 72]. The fact that the anterior segment AS-OCT provides in vivo information that cannot be obtained with videokeratoscopy and standard methods in CL applications of KC patients has led to an increasing interest in AS-OCT in CL practitioners. AS-OCT helps to examine the corneal midperiphery, the limbus region, the border structure of CL [73, 74]. Although OCT can also help evaluate scleral curvature, which will be useful in peripheral designs of S-CLs, it is not yet possible to measure scleral shape. OCT also helps to accurately evaluate the interaction between the anterior corneal and conjuctival surface and CL (**Figure 3**). It can measure the central and peripheral tear film clearance under the CL and thus provides information about the fitting [75, 76]. Central and peripheral vaults of hybrid, scleral and miniscleral lenses can also be measured with OCT. This helps us to examine in detail the relationship between asymmetric cornea and CL in KC. With using AS-OCT in CL practice, the maximum central cone vault values required to prevent edema due to hypoxia in the cornea under the scleral lens have been suggested. OCT also plays a major role in defining the relationship between CL and tears [8, 77].

4. Conclusions

Despite current surgical advances in KC treatment, CLs continue to be important for visual rehabilitation (even after surgery) in KC. Advances in CL design and materials have significantly expanded the application area of CL in the KC and ensured that the majority of patients have a satisfactory visual acuity. Thus, the rate of patients undergoing keratoplasty has decreased or the need for keratoplasty has been delayed. Although it takes a lot of time to choose the appropriate lens in KC, most of the patients with KC can benefit from CL use with the new designs and materials developed. CLs offer non-surgical options generally preferred for vision rehabilitation in the KC. SCLs, RGPs, PBCLs, HCLs, S-CLs constitute the contemporary range of lens types available for the vision rehabilitation of KC patients. This wide CL range meets the optometric needs of most of the patients with KC disease today and eliminates the need for major surgical procedures such as keratoplasty for vision rehabilitation for most of the patients.

Today, while SCL and HCL are the most commonly used in mild KC, the most frequently used CL in advanced KC is still RGPs and S-CLs. Since KC is a progressive disease, CL compliance should be controlled dynamically in certain periods of the patient's vision and comfort. If discomfort or intolerance develops in RGP, soft toric, PBCL or hybrid lenses may be considered. In the initial stages of the disease, SCLs are usually applied before other CLs are tried. Thus, the patient attains a good visual acuity and quality of life. When SCLs cannot provide this, secondly, RGPs are preferred because they provide a significant improvement in vision quality. When unsuccessful results are obtained with these CLs, PBCL or HCLs are used. If problems are encountered with these CLs, S-CLs are usually tried before surgery as a last option.

Imaging technologies such as corneal topography and OCT have enabled us to examine in vivo the relationship between asymmetric cornea and lens in the KC. Even with different modern CL treatments, it was found that both the quality of vision and life were lower in KC patients compared with the control group (healthy individuals without KC disease). This shows that CL treatment options and alternatives in KC treatment still need to be advanced.

Conflict of interest

The authors declare no conflict of interest.

Author details

Ersin Muhafiz
Kafkas University Faculty of Medicine, Kars, Turkey

*Address all correspondence to: ersinmuhafiz@hotmail.com

References

[1] Serdarogullari H, Tetikoglu M, Karahan H, Altin F, Elcioglu M. Prevalence of keratoconus and subclinical keratoconus in subjects with astigmatism using pentacam derived parameters. J Ophthalmic Vis Res 2013; 8(3): 213-9.

[2] Moschos MM, Nitoda E, Georgoudis P, Balidis M, Karageorgiadis E, Kozeis N. Contact lenses for keratoconus- current practice. Open Ophthalmol J. 2017;**11**:241-251. DOI: 10.2174/1874364101711010241

[3] Tan JCK, Nguyen V, Fenwick E, Ferdi A, Dinh A, Watson SL. Vision related quality of life in keratoconus: A save sight keratoconus registry study. Cornea. 2019;**38**(5):600-604. DOI: 10.1097/ICO.0000000000001899

[4] Kankariya VP, Kymionis GD, Diakonis VF, Yoo SH. Management of pediatric keratoconus - evolving role of corneal collagen cross-linking: An update. Indian Journal of Ophthalmology. 2013;**61**:435-440. DOI: 10.4103/0301-4738.116070

[5] Bozkurt E, Ucak T. Serum inflammation biomarkers in patients with keratoconus. Ocular Immunology and Inflammation. 2020:1-4. DOI: 10.1080/09273948.2020.1741648

[6] Bozkurt E, Bagcier F. Keratoconus: a potential risk factor for osteoarthritis. Int Ophthalmol. 2020;10.1007/s10792-020-01434-0. doi:10.1007/s10792-020-01434-0

[7] Shetty R, Kaweri L, Pahuja N, et al. Current review and a simplified "five-point management algorithm" for keratoconus. Indian Journal of Ophthalmology. 2015;**63**(1):46-53. DOI: 10.4103/0301-4738.151468

[8] Şengör T, Aydın Kurna S. Update on contact lens treatment of keratoconus. Turk J Ophthalmol. 2020;**50**(4):234-244. DOI: 10.4274/tjo.galenos.2020.70481

[9] Muhafiz E, Bayhan HA, Şahin S, Göçmen AY, Aslan Bayhan S, Gürdal C. Evaluation of the ocular surface in different contact lens replacement schedules. Cornea. 2019;**38**(5):587-594. DOI: 10.1097/ICO.0000000000001870

[10] Marsack JD, Ravikumar A, Nguyen C, Ticak A, Koenig DE, Elswick JD, et al. Wavefront-guided scleral lens correction in keratoconus. Optometry and Vision Science. 2014;**91**:1221-1230. DOI: 10.1097/OPX.0000000000000275

[11] Lim L, Lim EWL. Current perspectives in the management of keratoconus with contact lenses [published online ahead of print, 2020 Jul 8]. Eye (Lond). 2020;10.1038/s41433-020-1065-z. doi:10.1038/s41433-020-1065-z

[12] Rico-Del-Viejo L, Garcia-Montero M, Hernández-Verdejo JL, García-Lázaro S, Gómez-Sanz FJ, Lorente-Velázquez A. Nonsurgical procedures for keratoconus management. Journal of Ophthalmology 2017;2017:9707650. doi:10.1155/2017/9707650

[13] Rathi VM, Mandathara PS, Dumpati S. Contact lens in keratoconus. Indian Journal of Ophthalmology. 2013;**61**(8):410-415. DOI: 10.4103/0301-4738.116066

[14] Weed KH, MacEwen CJ, Giles T, Low J, McGhee CN. The Dundee university Scottish keratoconus study: Demographics, corneal signs, associated diseases, and eye rubbing. Eye (London, England). 2008;**22**(4):534-541. DOI: 10.1038/sj.eye.6702692

[15] Sultan P, Dogan C, Iskeleli G. A retrospective analysis of vision

correction and safety in keratoconus patients wearing Toris K soft contact lenses. International Ophthalmology. 2016;**36**(6):799-805. DOI: 10.1007/s10792-016-0200-0

[16] Yildiz EH, Erdurmus M, Elibol ES, Acar B, Vural ET. Contact lens impact on quality of life in keratoconus patients: Rigid gas permeable versus soft silicone-hydrogel keratoconus lenses. International Journal of Ophthalmology. 2015;**8**(5):1074-1077. DOI: 10.3980/j.issn.2222-3959.2015.05.38

[17] Jinabhai A, O'Donnell C, Tromans C, Radhakrishnan H. Optical quality and visual performance with customised soft contact lenses for keratoconus. Ophthalmic & Physiological Optics. 2014;**34**(5):528-539. DOI: 10.1111/opo.12133

[18] Gumus K, Kahraman N. A new fitting approach for providing adequate comfort and visual performance in keratoconus: Soft HydroCone (Toris K) lenses. Eye & Contact Lens. 2016;**42**(4):225-230. DOI: 10.1097/ICL.0000000000000183

[19] Fernandez-Velazquez FJ. Kerasoft IC compared to rose-K in the management of corneal ectasias. Contact Lens & Anterior Eye. 2012;**35**(4):175-179. DOI: 10.1016/j.clae.2012.02.005

[20] Carballo-Alvarez J, Puell MC, Cuiña R, Diaz-Valle D, Vazquez JM, Benitez-Del-Castillo JM. Soft contact lens fitting after intrastromal corneal ring segment implantation to treat keratoconus. Contact Lens & Anterior Eye. 2014;**37**(5):377-381. DOI: 10.1016/j.clae.2014.06.001

[21] de Brabander J, Chateau N, Marin G, Lopez-Gil N, Van Der Worp E, Benito A. Simulated optical performance of custom wavefront soft contact lenses for keratoconus. Optometry and Vision Science. 2003;**80**(9):637-643. DOI: 10.1097/00006324-200309000-00008

[22] Bilgin LK, Yilmaz S, Araz B, Yüksel SB, Sezen T. 30 years of contact lens prescribing for keratoconic patients in Turkey. Contact Lens & Anterior Eye. 2009;**32**(1):16-21. DOI: 10.1016/j.clae.2008.07.001

[23] Downie LE, Lindsay RG. Contact lens management of keratoconus. Clinical & Experimental Optometry. 2015;**98**(4):299-311. DOI: 10.1111/cxo.12300

[24] Weed KH, Macewen CJ, McGhee CN. The Dundee university Scottish keratoconus study II: A prospective study of optical and surgical correction. Ophthalmic & Physiological Optics. 2007;**27**:561-567

[25] Yazar E, Alaçayır F, Asyalı Altınok A, Kurtuluş S, Öztürk F. Results of application of rigid gas permeable contact lenses in patients with keratoconus. Turk J Ophthalmol. 2013;**43**:432-436

[26] Araki S, Koh S, Kabata D, et al. Effect of long-term rigid gas-permeable contact lens wear on keratoconus progression. The British Journal of Ophthalmology 2020;bjophthalmol-2020-315942. doi:10.1136/bjophthalmol-2020-315942

[27] Gumus K, Gire A, Pflugfelder SC. The impact of the Boston ocular surface prosthesis on wavefront higher-order aberrations. American Journal of Ophthalmology. 2011;**151**(4):682-690.e2. DOI: 10.1016/j.ajo.2010.10.027

[28] López-Gil N, Castejón-Mochón JF, Fernández-Sánchez V. Limitations of the ocular wavefront correction with contact lenses. Vision Research. 2009;**49**(14):1729-1737. DOI: 10.1016/j.visres.2009.04.016

[29] Negishi K, Kumanomido T, Utsumi Y, Tsubota K. Effect of higher-order aberrations on visual function in keratoconic eyes with

a rigid gas permeable contact lens. American Journal of Ophthalmology. 2007;**144**(6):924-929. DOI: 10.1016/j.ajo.2007.08.004

[30] Korb DR, Finnemore VM, Herman JP. Apical changes and scarring in keratoconus as related to contact lens fitting techniques. Journal of the American Optometric Association. 1982;**53**:199-205

[31] Leung KKY. RGP fitting philosophies for keratoconus. Clinical & Experimental Optometry. 1999;**82**:230-235

[32] Mandell RB. Contemporary management of keratoconus. Int Contact Lens Clin. 1997;**24**:43-55

[33] Lunardi LH, Arroyo D, Andrade Sobrinho MV, Lipener C, Rosa JM. Descriptive analysis of the type and design of contact lenses fitted according to keratoconus severity and morphology. Arquivos Brasileiros de Oftalmologia. 2016;**79**(2):82-84. DOI: 10.5935/0004-2749.20160025

[34] Wilson SE, Lin DT, Klyce SD, Reidy JJ, Insler MS. Rigid contact lens decentration: A risk factor for corneal warpage. The CLAO Journal. 1990;**16**(3):177-182

[35] Wagner H, Barr JT, Zadnik K. Collaborative longitudinal evaluation of keratoconus (CLEK) study: Methods and findings to date. Contact Lens & Anterior Eye. 2007;**30**(4):223-232. DOI: 10.1016/j.clae.2007.03.001

[36] Edrington TB, Gundel RE, Libassi DP, et al. Variables affecting rigid contact lens comfort in the collaborative longitudinal evaluation of keratoconus (CLEK) study. Optometry and Vision Science. 2004;**81**(3):182-188. DOI: 10.1097/00006324-200403000-00010

[37] Wu Y, Tan Q, Zhang W, et al. Rigid gas-permeable contact lens related life quality in keratoconic patients with different grades of severity. Clinical & Experimental Optometry. 2015;**98**(2):150-154. DOI: 10.1111/cxo.12237

[38] Güneş a, Kubaloğlu A, Bayramlar H. Rose K lenses for keratoconus. Turk J Ophthalmol 2012; 42: 88-90.

[39] Carracedo G, González-Méijome JM, Martín-Gil A, Carballo J, Pintor J. The influence of rigid gas permeable lens wear on the concentrations of dinucleotides in tears and the effect on dry eye signs and symptoms in keratoconus. Contact Lens & Anterior Eye 2016 39(5):375-379. doi:10.1016/j.clae.2016.04.009

[40] Huang T, Hu Y, Gui M, Zhang H, Wang Y, Hou C. Large-diameter deep anterior lamellar keratoplasty for keratoconus: Visual and refractive outcomes. The British Journal of Ophthalmology. 2015;**99**(9):1196-1200. DOI: 10.1136/bjophthalmol-2014-306170

[41] Zadnik K, Barr JT, Edrington TB, et al. Baseline findings in the collaborative longitudinal evaluation of keratoconus (CLEK) study. Investigative Ophthalmology & Visual Science. 1998;**39**(13):2537-2546

[42] Uçakhan OO, Kanpolat A, Ozdemir O. Contact lens fitting for keratoconus after Intacs placement. Eye & Contact Lens. 2006;**32**(2):75-77. DOI: 10.1097/01.icl.0000174749.96423.ca

[43] Barnett M, Mannis MJ. Contact lenses in the management of keratoconus. Cornea. 2011;**30**(12):1510-1516. DOI: 10.1097/ICO.0b013e318211401f

[44] Michaud L, Brazeau D, Corbeil ME, Forcier P, Bernard PJ. Contribution of soft lenses of various powers to the optics of a piggy-back system on regular

corneas. Contact Lens & Anterior Eye. 2013;**36**(6):318-323. DOI: 10.1016/j.clae.2013.02.005

[45] Romero-Jiménez M, Santodomingo-Rubido J, Flores-Rodríguez P, González-Méijome JM. Which soft contact lens power is better for piggyback fitting in keratoconus? Contact Lens & Anterior Eye. 2013;**36**(1):45-48. DOI: 10.1016/j.clae.2012.10.070

[46] Acar BT, Vural ET, Acar S. Effects of contact lenses on the ocular surface in patients with keratoconus: Piggyback versus ClearKone hybrid lenses. Eye & Contact Lens. 2012;**38**(1):43-48. DOI: 10.1097/ICL.0b013e31823ff181

[47] López-Alemany A, González-Méijome JM, Almeida JB, Parafita MA, Refojo MF. Oxygen transmissibility of piggyback systems with conventional soft and silicone hydrogel contact lenses. Cornea. 2006;**25**(2):214-219. DOI: 10.1097/01.ico.0000178276.90892.ac

[48] Sengor T, Kurna SA, Aki S, Ozkurt Y. High Dk piggyback contact lens system for contact lens-intolerant keratoconus patients. Clinical Ophthalmology. 2011;**5**:331-335. DOI: 10.2147/OPTH.S16727

[49] Nau AC. A comparison of synergeyes versus traditional rigid gas permeable lens designs for patients with irregular corneas. Eye & Contact Lens. 2008;**34**(4):198-200. DOI: 10.1097/ICL.0b013e31815c859b

[50] Altay Y, Balta O, Burcu A, Ornek F. Hybrid contact lenses for visual management of patients after keratoplasty. Nigerian Journal of Clinical Practice. 2018;**21**(4):451-455. DOI: 10.4103/njcp.njcp_103_17

[51] Hassani M, Jafarzadehpur E, Mirzajani A, Yekta A. Khabazkhoob M. a comparison of the visual acuity outcome between Clearkone and RGP lenses. J Curr Ophthalmol. 2017;**30**(1):85-86. DOI: 10.1016/j.joco.2017.08.006

[52] Abdalla YF, Elsahn AF, Hammersmith KM, Cohen EJ. SynergEyes lenses for keratoconus. Cornea. 2010;**29**(1):5-8. DOI: 10.1097/ICO.0b013e3181a9d090

[53] Pullum KW, Whiting MA, Buckley RJ. Scleral contact lenses: The expanding role. Cornea. 2005;**24**(3):269-277. DOI: 10.1097/01.ico.0000148311.94180.6b

[54] Rathi VM, Mandathara PS, Taneja M, Dumpati S, Sangwan VS. Scleral lens for keratoconus: Technology update. Clinical Ophthalmology. 2015;**9**:2013-2018. DOI: 10.2147/OPTH.S52483

[55] Jaynes JM, Edrington TB, Weissman BA. Predicting scleral GP lens entrapped tear layer oxygen tensions. Contact Lens & Anterior Eye. 2015;**38**(1):44-47. DOI: 10.1016/j.clae.2014.09.008

[56] Visser ES, Visser R, Van Lier HJ. Advantages of toric scleral lenses. Optometry and Vision Science. 2006;**83**(4):233-236. DOI: 10.1097/01.opx.0000214297.38421.15

[57] Vincent SJ, Fadel D. Optical considerations for scleral contact lenses: A review. Contact Lens & Anterior Eye. 2019;**42**(6):598-613. DOI: 10.1016/j.clae.2019.04.012

[58] Hussoin T, Le HG, Carrasquillo KG, Johns L, Rosenthal P, Jacobs DS. The effect of optic asphericity on visual rehabilitation of corneal ectasia with a prosthetic device. Eye & Contact Lens. 2012;**38**(5):300-305. DOI: 10.1097/ICL.0b013e3182657da5

[59] Schornack MM, Patel SV. Scleral lenses in the management of keratoconus. Eye & Contact Lens. 2010;**36**(1):39-44. DOI: 10.1097/ICL.0b013e3181c786a6

[60] Alipour F, Kheirkhah A, Jabarvand Behrouz M. Use of mini scleral contact lenses in moderate to severe dry eye. Contact Lens & Anterior Eye. 2012;**35**(6):272-276. DOI: 10.1016/j.clae.2012.07.006

[61] Visser ES, Soeters N, Tahzib NG. Scleral lens tolerance after corneal cross-linking for keratoconus. Optometry and Vision Science. 2015;**92**(3):318-323. DOI: 10.1097/OPX.0000000000000515

[62] Alipour F, Rahimi F, Hashemian MN, Ajdarkosh Z, Roohipoor R, Mohebi M. Mini-scleral contact lens for Management of Poor Visual Outcomes after intrastromal corneal ring segments implantation in keratoconus. J. Ophthalmic Vis. Res. 2016;**11**(3):252-257. DOI: 10.4103/2008-322X.188400

[63] Barnett M, Lien V, Li JY, Durbin-Johnson B, Mannis MJ. Use of scleral lenses and Miniscleral lenses after penetrating Keratoplasty. Eye & Contact Lens. 2016;**42**(3):185-189. DOI: 10.1097/ICL.0000000000000163

[64] Rathi VM, Mandathara PS, Vaddavalli PK, Srikanth D, Sangwan VS. Fluid filled scleral contact lens in pediatric patients: Challenges and outcome. Contact Lens & Anterior Eye. 2012;**35**(4):189-192. DOI: 10.1016/j.clae.2012.03.001

[65] Koppen C, Kreps EO, Anthonissen L, Van Hoey M, Dhubhghaill SN, Vermeulen L. Scleral lenses reduce the need for corneal transplants in severe keratoconus. American Journal of Ophthalmology. 2018;**185**:43-47. DOI: 10.1016/j.ajo.2017.10.022

[66] Bergmanson JP, Walker MK, Johnson LA. Assessing scleral contact lens satisfaction in a keratoconus population. Optometry and Vision Science. 2016;**93**(8):855-860. DOI: 10.1097/OPX.0000000000000882

[67] Bruce AS, Nguyen LM. Acute red eye (non-ulcerative keratitis) associated with mini-scleral contact lens wear for keratoconus. Clinical & Experimental Optometry. 2013;**96**(2):245-248. DOI: 10.1111/cxo.12033

[68] Zimmerman AB, Marks A. Microbial keratitis secondary to unintended poor compliance with scleral gas-permeable contact lenses. Eye & Contact Lens. 2014;**40**(1):e1-e4. DOI: 10.1097/ICL.0b013e318273420f

[69] Sorbara L, Dalton K. The use of video-keratoscopy in predicting contact lens parameters for keratoconic fitting. Contact Lens & Anterior Eye. 2010;**33**(3):112-118. DOI: 10.1016/j.clae.2010.01.002

[70] Downie LE. Predictive value of corneal topography for ClearKone hybrid contact lenses. Optometry and Vision Science. 2013;**90**(7):e191-e197. DOI: 10.1097/OPX.0b013e318297da25

[71] Nosch DS, Ong GL, Mavrikakis I, Morris J. The application of a computerised videokeratography (CVK) based contact lens fitting software programme on irregularly shaped corneal surfaces. Contact Lens & Anterior Eye. 2007;**30**(4):239-248. DOI: 10.1016/j.clae.2007.06.003

[72] Sonsino J, Mathe DS. Central vault in dry eye patients successfully wearing scleral lens. Optometry and Vision Science. 2013;**90**(9):e248-e1030. DOI: 10.1097/OPX.0000000000000013

[73] Luo ZK, Jacobs DS. Current and potential applications of anterior segment optical coherence tomography in contact lens fitting. Seminars in Ophthalmology. 2012;**27**(5-6):133-137. DOI: 10.3109/08820538.2012.708814

[74] Wolffsohn JS, Drew T, Dhallu S, Sheppard A, Hofmann GJ, Prince M. Impact of soft contact lens edge design and midperipheral lens shape on the epithelium and its indentation with lens mobility. Investigative Ophthalmology & Visual Science. 2013;**54**(9):6190-6197. DOI: 10.1167/iovs.13-12425

[75] Choi HJ, Lee SM, Lee JY, Lee SY, Kim MK, Wee WR. Measurement of anterior scleral curvature using anterior segment OCT. Optometry and Vision Science. 2014;**91**(7):793-802. DOI: 10.1097/OPX.0000000000000298

[76] Elbendary AM, Abou Samra W. Evaluation of rigid gas permeable lens fitting in keratoconic patients with optical coherence tomography. Graefe's Archive for Clinical and Experimental Ophthalmology. 2013;**251**(6):1565-1570. DOI: 10.1007/s00417-013-2271-1

[77] Michaud L, van der Worp E, Brazeau D, Warde R, Giasson CJ. Predicting estimates of oxygen transmissibility for scleral lenses. Contact Lens & Anterior Eye. 2012;**35**(6):266-271. DOI: 10.1016/j.clae.2012.07.004

Chapter 5

Geometric Analysis of Ophthalmic Lens by Backward Method and Optical Simulation

Rung-Sheng Chen

Abstract

This chapter will show the optical models of ametropia and presyopia by backward method (BM). The design activity of ophthalmic lens involves relatively simple, often elementary geometric optics. In general, ophthalmic lens design is given by tracing the light from the object to the image plane, i.e., the retina. And this can be called the forward method (AM). By BM, the position of the object and image is interchanged, i.e., retina plays the role as object. Using BM gives an alternative way to know how the eye works as a lens, and the retina now acts as the object tells more information for the correction of ametropia and presbyopia for its curve shape and the location. Applying this BM geometric analysis, we can see the correction of ametropia by correction lens, i.e., spectacle, is to fulfill the needs to put the object at the conjugate places of retina formed by the myopic and hyperopic eye. For verification, the optical simulation by Zemax is applied to simulate the image forming processing, i.e., the conjugation between the retinal and it counter parts. Similarly, this geometric analysis can be applied to analyze the progressive addition lenses (PALs) by the revised BM.

Keywords: geometry optics, ophthalmic lens, ametropia, presyopia, simulation

1. Introduction

In general, optical image forming is to trace light ray from object to image shown in **Figure 1**, i.e., from the left to the right which represents the object and image spaces respectively [1, 2]. And this can be called the forward method (FM). This chapter shows that the retinal of the eye plays the role as the object, and the light ray is traced from the right to the left compared to the FM. Since the ray racing is formed from the right to the left, i.e., backward method, this is named as BM. By BM, it will be analytically examined the ametropia and presbyopia.

At retinal, its edge zones in curved facing to object with closer distance compared with the central zone. In BM, it traces the light in an offense controversial way as the retinal acts now as the object rather than an image as usual. Using BM, it gives another way to look after how human's eye traces the light from the object to sit at the retina. But now, light rays emerge from the retinal is traced to the image plane where is at infinity as emmetropia or at the designated one as ametropia. Applying this unconventional geometry analysis, we can see the correction of ametropia by correction lens, i.e., spectacle, is to fulfill the needs to put the object at the

IntechOpen

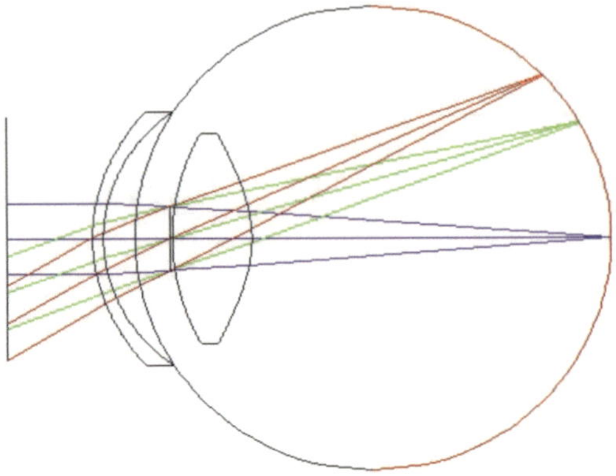

Figure 1.
Forward method of retinal image forming of emmetropic eye with field angle varied by 0, 20, and 30°.

conjugate places of the retina formed by the myopic and hyperopic eye [3]. Similarly, this geometric analysis will be applied to analyze the progressive addition lenses (PALs) [4] by the revised BM.

As mentioned in the fundamental infrastructure of the object and image layout [1]. The location and size of the image formed by a given optical system can be determined by locating the respective images of the sources making up the object. Here **Figure 2** shows the methodology of backward method of retinal imaging forming of emmetropic eye.

Figure 1 shows the conventional forward method of retinal image forming where retinal serves as the image. And **Figure 2** shows the backward method of retinal image forming where retinal serves as an object. By the BM idea, the object distance is finite and its shape is curve rather than plane, this can be an alternative way to realize the way of image forming by emmetropic or ametropic eye.

The following sections will give a rigorous analysis of BM, and the optical simulation by Zemax will accompanied for ophthalmic lens maker to have a clue to design a suitable spectacle for the glass wear. The data sheets of emmetropic eye are shown in **Tables 1** and **2** which represented the construction data of FM and BM of emmetropic eye.

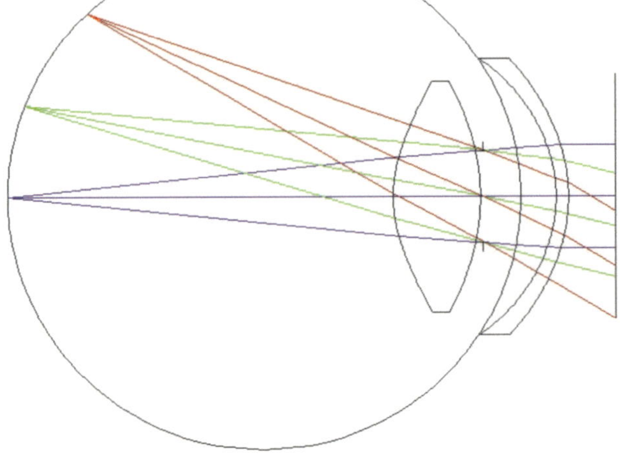

Figure 2.
Backward method of retinal image forming of emmetropic eye with object height varied by 0, 4, and 8 mm.

Surf: type		Comment	Radius	Thickness	Glass	Semi-diameter		Conic
*	Standard		Infinity	Infinity		Infinity	U	0.000
1	Standard		Infinity	4.000		5.764		0.000
2*	Standard	Cornea	7.800	0.520	Cornea	6.000	U	−0.500
3*	Standard		6.700	1.500	Aqueous	6.000	U	−0.300
4	Standard		11.000	1.600	Aqueous	11.000	U	0.000
*	Standard	Pupil	Infinity	0.100	Aqueous	1.500	U	0.000
6*	Standard	Lens	10.000	3.700	Lens	5.000	U	0.000
7*	Standard		−6.000	16.580	Vitreous	5.000	U	−3.250
IMA	Standard	Retina	−11.000	—	Vitreous	11.000	U	0.000

When an aperture is defined on a surface, ZEMAX will display an asterisk "" symbol next to the surface number.*

Table 1.
*Optical data of forward method of retinal image forming of emmetropic eye (*next to the surface number means an aperture is defined on this surface).*

Surf: type		Comment	Radius	Thickness	Glass	Semi-diameter		Conic
*	Standard	Retina	11.000	16.580	Vitreous	8.000		0.000
1*	Standard	Lens	6.000	3.700	Lens	5.000	U	−3.000
2*	Standard		−10.000	0.100	Aqueous	5.000	U	0.000
STO	Standard	Pupil	Infinity	1.600	Aqueous	2.000	U	0.000
4	Standard		−11.000	1.500	Aqueous	11.000	U	0.000
5*	Standard	Cornea	−6.700	0.520	Cornea	6.000	U	−0.300
6*	Standard	Subject eye	−7.800	2.000		6.000	U	−0.500
IMA	Standard		Infinity	—		5.340		0.000

When an aperture is defined on a surface, ZEMAX will display an asterisk "" symbol next to the surface number.*

Table 2.
Optical data of backward method of retinal image forming of emmetropic eye.

2. Geometric analysis of ametropia

The function of ophthalmic lens to correct vision can be analysis on the basis of elementary of geometry. In geometric analysis, an object and the image of the object created by any optical system are said to be conjugate to one another. In a nonaccommodating emmetropic eye, a distant object is focus on the retina as shown in **Figure 1**.

2.1 Myopia

If the eyes' optical elements do not create conjugant between the retina and a distance object, ametropia exists. In the myopic eye, the image of a distant object is not on the retina but located in front of it. **Figure 3** shows an −10 D myopic eye whose axial distance is 20.28 mm compared with 16.58 mm of emmetropic one shown in **Table 1**, as eye axis increases by 0.37 mm, the diopter of the myopic eye increases by −1.00 D [5].

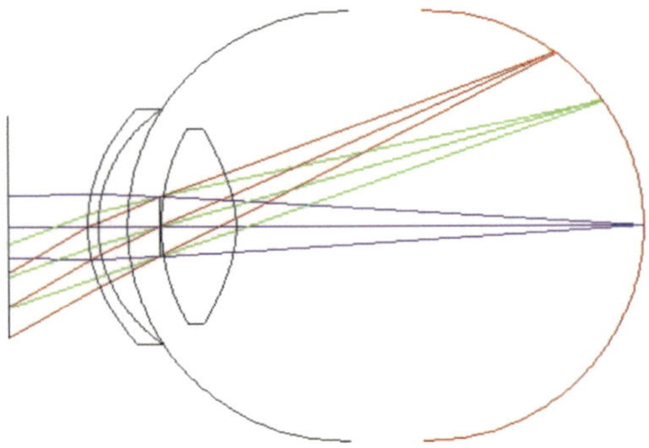

Figure 3.
Layout of −10 D myopic eye.

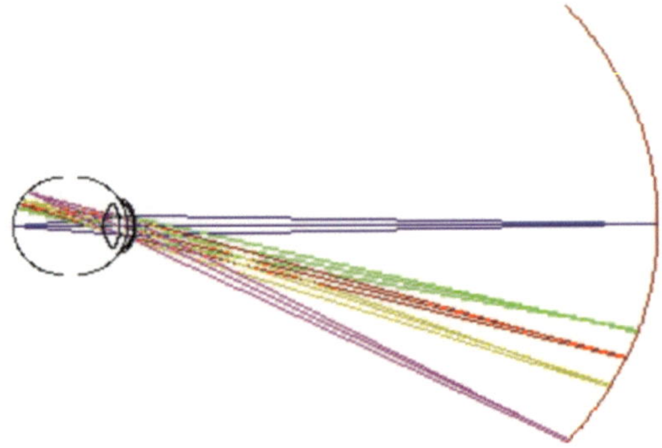

Figure 4.
−10 D myopia ray trace form optical simulation by BM.

If the retina of an eye is thought by BM as an object, the image of the retina formed by the optics of Eye will be located at the far point plane [6], i.e., the conjugate plane of the retina. Following the backward method (BM), in the emmetropic eye, the far point plane is located at optical infinity as shown in **Figure 2**. But in the myopic eye, the far point plane is not located at infinity but somewhere in front of the eye. And this can be simulated by optical simulation by Zemax shown in **Figure 4**.

This can also be explained graphically as the retina is located at a bit longer distance than the focal length of the myopic eye. The far point plane is real, inverted, and relative huge. And the higher the degree of myopia, the closer the far point plane is to the eye as shown in **Figures 5** and **6**.

This can be explained by "Newtonian" form of the image Eq. (1), we can see:

$$x' = -\frac{f^2}{x} \tag{1}$$

where x and x' are the distances from focal point to the object and image, respectively, and f is the focal length of the optics of eye.

In the case of lower degree of myopia, it means the retina is in front of the focal point of the optics of eye, i.e., $x < 0$, and $x \cong 0$. Keep in mind, the sign is still valid in an alternative way by BM. From Eq. (1), we can see the conjugant image distance is real, i.e., $x' > 0$, and inverted, indicated by **Figures 5–8**.

Optical simulation by BM can also verify this phenomenon as illustrated in **Figures 7** and **8**, with −5 and −10 D myopia, respectively.

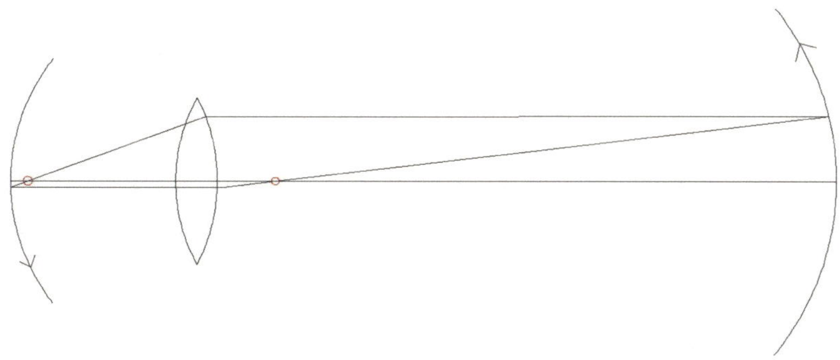

Figure 5.
Far point plane of low degree myopic eye. It is real, inverted, and relatively huge.

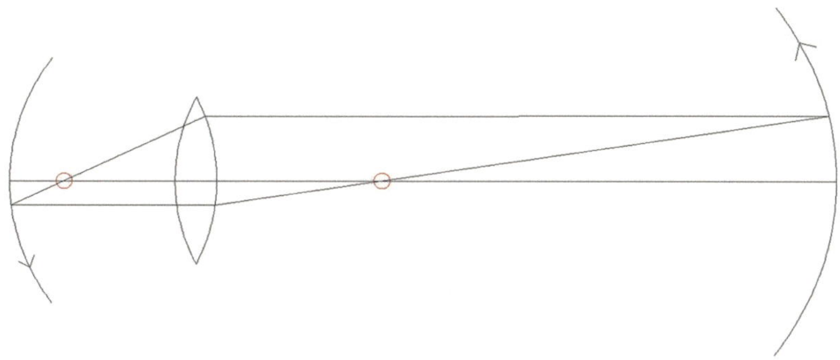

Figure 6.
Far point plane of high degree myopic eye.

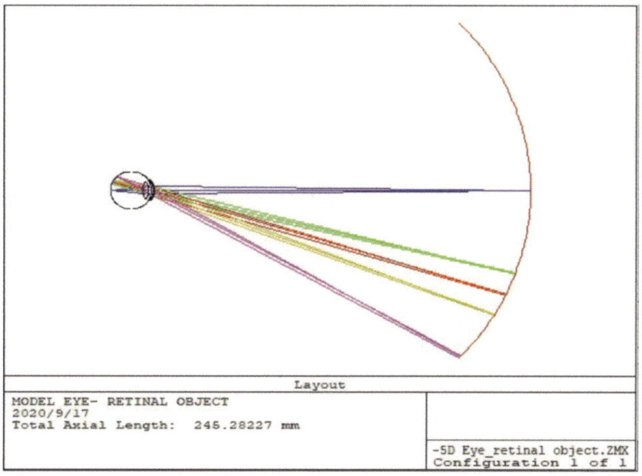

Figure 7.
Ray tracing of −5 D myopic eye by BM.

The magnification of the image of the retina is determined by Eq. (2):

$$m = \frac{f}{x} \tag{2}$$

This means the image size of the retina is relatively huge as $x \cong 0$. And this shows the reason why an emmetropic or lower degree of myopia can look easily the

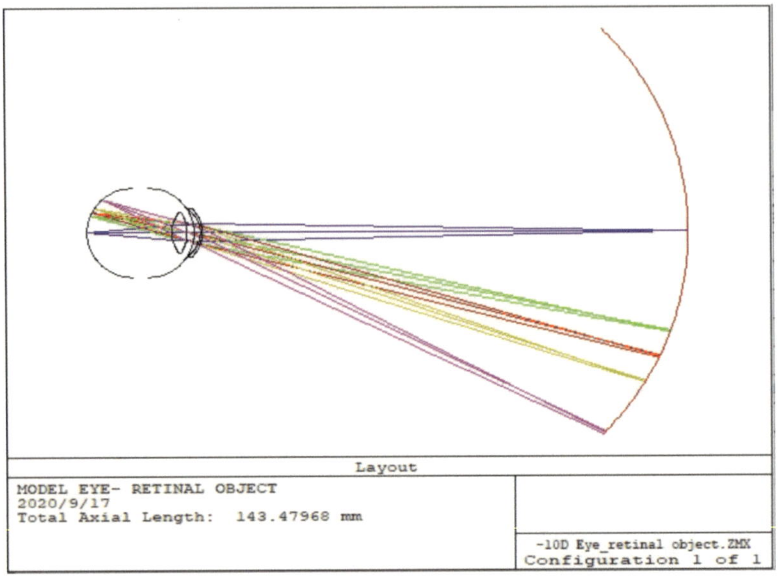

Figure 8.
Ray tracing of −10 D myopic eye by BM.

sightseeing because the image plane of the retina is approximately as a plain with relatively large scale. As the degree of myopia is increased, i.e., x is getting longer, the image size of the retina is decreased by Eq. (2) as m is inverse proportional to x. This makes the field of view of high degree myopia be restricted to a relative small scale. The optical simulation proves this shown in **Tables 3** and **4**.

Concerning the image quality of BM of myopic eye ray trace, we can also see an interesting phenomenon indicating the distortion changed with the curvature of the image plane of the retina, i.e., the shape of viewing object. **Figures 9** and **10** show the scale of the curvature of the retina's image decreased from −140 to −70 mm to get a corrected undistorted image, i.e., distortion ≒ 0.2%.

From the above discussion, we can see that the scale and the curvature of the image plane changing from −5 to −10 D myopic eye are related to the factor of 2 as expected by Eq. (2). And Eq. (1) gives a clue to locate the places of far point plane; the thickness from eye to the image plane is 219.432 and 115.780 mm related to −5 and −10 D myopia, respectively.

Surf: type		Comment	Radius	Thickness		Glass	Semi-diameter		Conic
*	Standard	Retina	11.000	18.430		Vitreous	8.000		0.000
1*	Standard	Lens	6.000	3.700		Lens	5.000	U	−3.000
2*	Standard		−10.000	0.100		Aqueous	5.000	U	0.000
STO	Standard	Pupil	Infinity	1.600		Aqueous	2.000	U	0.000
4	Standard		−11.000	1.500		Aqueous	11.000	U	0.000
5*	Standard	Cornea	−6.700	0.520		Cornea	6.000	U	−0.300
6*	Standard	Subject eye	−7.800	219.432	M		6.000	U	−0.500
IMA	Standard		−140.000	—			99.932		0.000

When an aperture is defined on a surface, ZEMAX will display an asterisk "" symbol next to the surface number.*

Table 3.
Optical data of −5 D myopic eye by BM (image semi-diameter: 99.932 mm).

Surf: type		Comment	Radius	Thickness		Glass	Semi-diameter		Conic
*	Standard	Retina	11.000	20.280		Vitreous	8.000		0.000
1*	Standard	Lens	6.000	3.700		Lens	5.000	U	−3.000
2*	Standard		−10.000	0.100		Aqueous	5.000	U	0.000
STO	Standard	Pupil	Infinity	1.600		Aqueous	2.000	U	0.000
4	Standard		−11.000	1.500		Aqueous	11.000	U	0.000
5*	Standard	Cornea	−6.700	0.520		Cornea	6.000	U	−0.300
6*	Standard	Subject eye	−7.800	115.780	M		6.000	U	−0.500
IMA	Standard		−70.000	—			45.389		0.000

When an aperture is defined on a surface, ZEMAX will display an asterisk "" symbol next to the surface number.*

Table 4.
Optical data of −10 D myopic eye by BM (image semi-diameter: 49.389 mm).

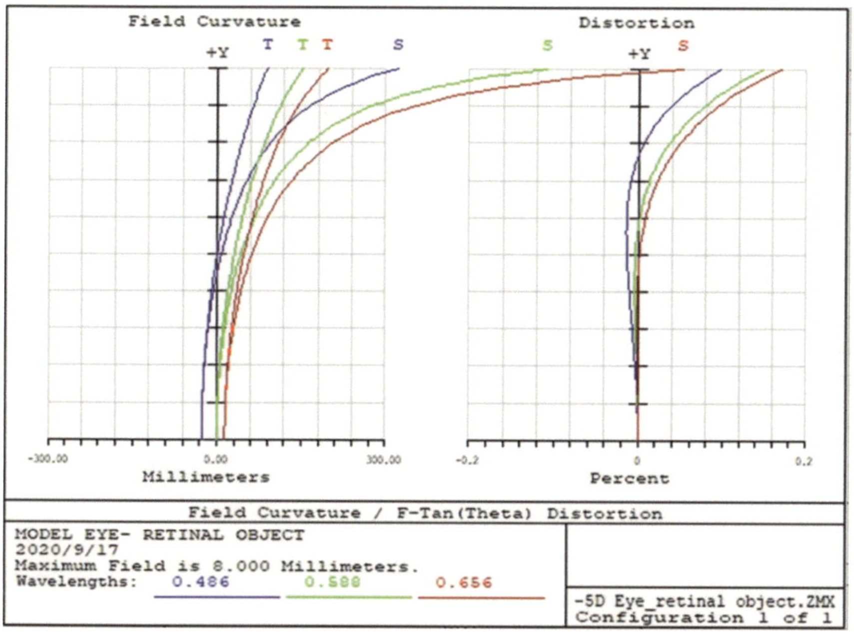

Figure 9.
Field curvature and distortion of −5 D myopic eye with corrected curvature of image plane of retina by BM.

The correction of myopia is to add the concave lens to let the distance object sit on the far point plane, and the design of the spectacle whose secondary focal plane is placed to coincide with the myopic eye's far point plane, as shown in **Figure 11** for the correction of −5 D myopia.

Table 5 shows the optical datasheet of −5 D myopia correction, and the object distance, object curvature, and object height are got from **Table 3** by BM.

We can see the spectacle is designed whose second focal point is coincide with the far point distance (219.432 mm), object's curvature is set by 140 mm, and the object height is 99.232 mm which is same as the image's semi-diameter in **Table 3**. Then the field curvature and distortion are well corrected by indication from **Figure 12**. It shows how BM can give a way to design an correction spectacle by finding the construction data from itself.

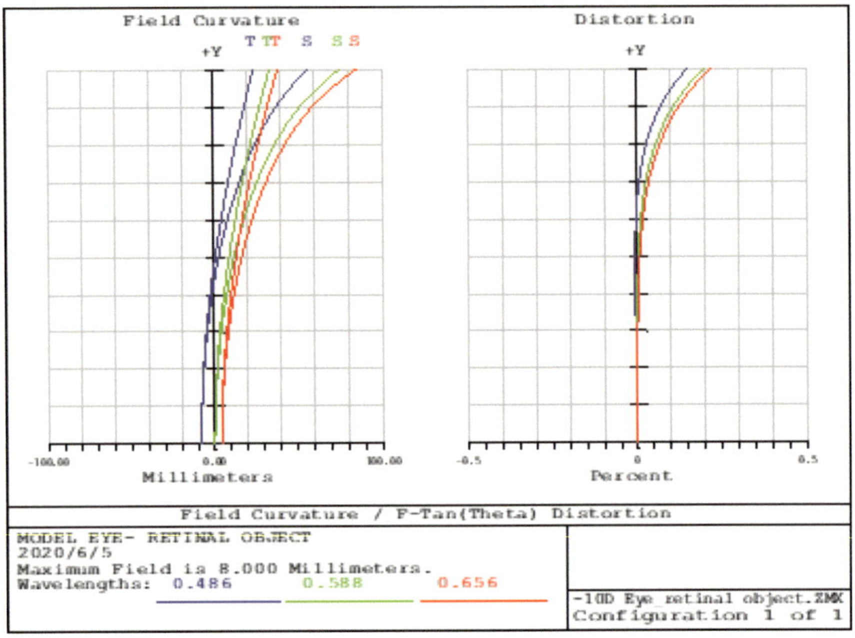

Figure 10.
Field curvature and distortion of −10 D myopic eye with corrected curvature of image plane of retina by BM.

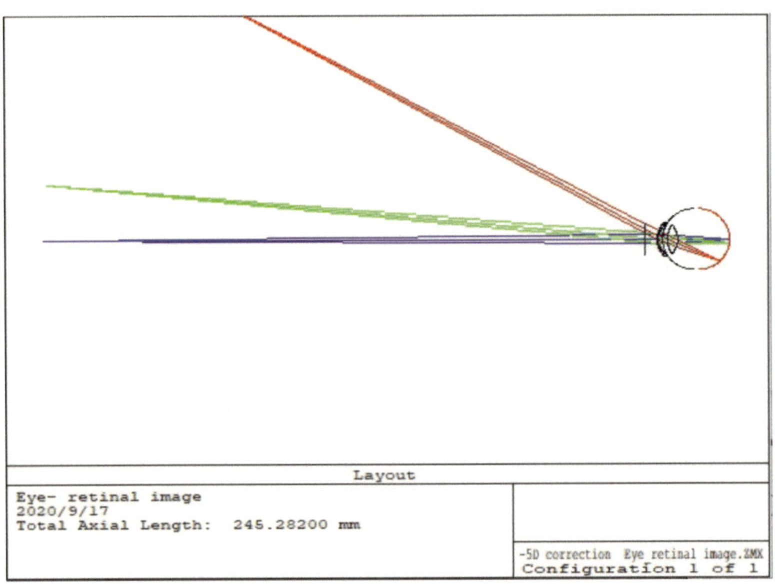

Figure 11.
Correction of −5 D myopia with 99.232 object height.

2.2 Hyperopia

In the hyperopic eye, the image of a distance object is not on the retina but located behind of it as shown in **Figure 13**.

In hyperopic eye, by BM the far point plane is virtual and located behind the eye in a virtual, erected, and relative large scale form because the retina is located at a bit shorter distance than the focal length of hyperopic eye. The higher degree of the

Surf: type		Comment	Radius	Thickness	Glass	Semi-diameter		Conic
*	Standard		140.000	215.432		0.000	U	0.000
1	Standard		Infinity	4.000		5.488		0.000
2*	Standard	Cornea	7.800	0.520	Cornea	6.000	U	−0.500
3*	Standard		6.700	1.500	Aqueous	6.000	U	−0.300
4	Standard		11.000	1.600	Aqueous	11.000	U	0.000
*	Standard	Pupil	Infinity	0.100	Aqueous	1.500	U	0.000
6*	Standard	Lens	10.000	3.700	Lens	5.000	U	0.000
7*	Standard		−6.000	18.430	Vitreous	5.000	U	−3.250
IMA	Standard	Retina	−11.000	—	Vitreous	11.000	U	0.000

When an aperture is defined on a surface, ZEMAX will display an asterisk "" symbol next to the surface number.*

Table 5.
Optical data of −5 D myopia correction.

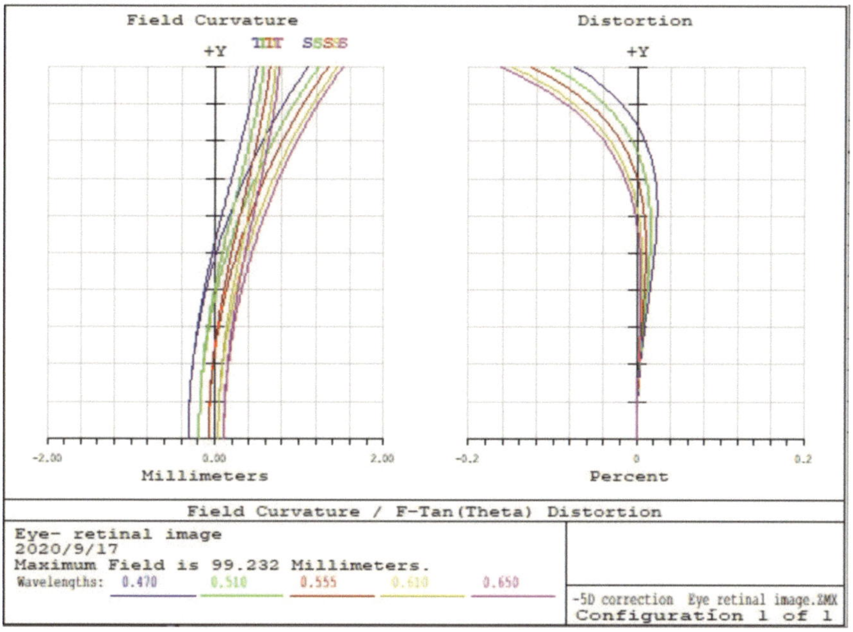

Figure 12.
*Field curvature and distortion of −5 D myopic eye with well correction by putting the far point at the designated data from **Table 3** by BM.*

hyperopia, the closer the far point plane is to the eye as shown in **Figures 14** and **15** and the **Tables 6** and 7 for the image distance changed from −178.364 to −83.003 mm respected with +5 to +10 D hyperopia.

The above optical simulation can also be graphically illustrated by **Figures 16** and **17**. It shows by using Eq. (1), we get $x' < 0$, and the far point plane which is the conjugant image of the retina is behind the eye as the retina is sit inside of the focal point of the optics of eye, i.e., $x > 0$.

The correction of hyperopia is to add the concave lens to let the distance object sit on the far point plane, and the design of the spectacle whose secondary focal plane is placed to coincide with the hyperopic eye's far point plane, as shown in **Figure 18** for the correction of +5 D myopia.

Table 8 shows the optical datasheet of +5 D hyperopia correction, and the object distance, object curvature, and object height are got from **Table 6** by BM.

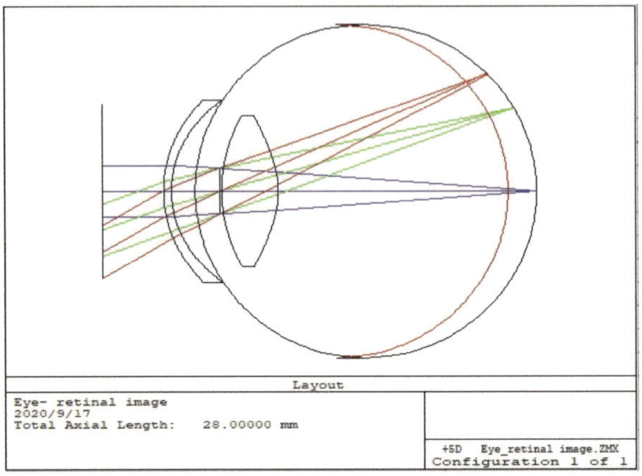

Figure 13.
+5 D hyperopic eye with 1.85 mm [5] shorter axial distance.

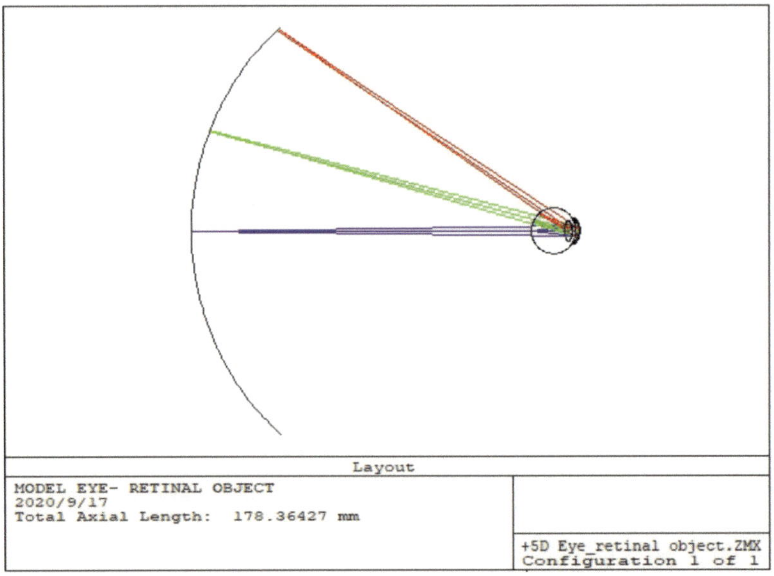

Figure 14.
Far point plane of +5 D hyperopic eye by BM.

We can see the spectacle is designed whose second focal point is coincide with the far point distance (−178.364 mm), object's curvature is set by −130 mm, and the object height is 94.996 mm which is same as the image's semi-diameter in **Table 3**. Then the field curvature and distortion are well corrected by indication from **Figure 19**. It shows how BM can give a way to design an correction spectacle by finding the construction data from itself.

3. Geometric analysis of presbyopia

The need to wear spectacles to see near objects is a result of presbyopia [7]. And this is different from the cases of hyperopia whose object is assumed at infinity. Presbyopia is a condition associated with aging in which the eye exhibits a progressively diminished ability to focus on near objects. Multifocal spectacle lenses or progressive addition lenses (PALs) are primarily used in the treatment of presbyopia [8].

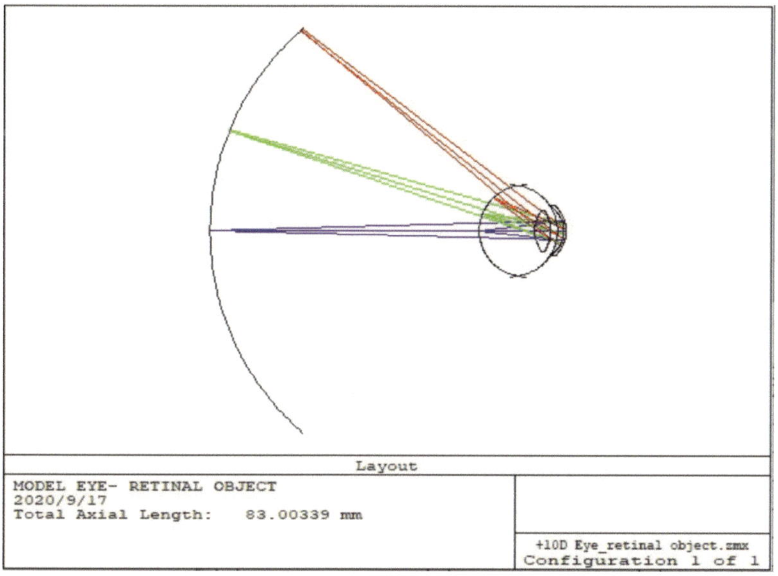

Figure 15.
Far point plane of +10 D hyperopic eye by BM.

Surf: type		Comment	Radius	Thickness		Glass	Semi-diameter		Conic
*	Standard	Retina	11.000	14.730		Vitreous	8.000		0.000
1*	Standard	Lens	6.000	3.700		Lens	5.000	U	−3.000
2*	Standard		−10.000	0.100		Aqueous	5.000	U	0.000
STO	Standard	Pupil	Infinity	1.600		Aqueous	2.000	U	0.000
4	Standard		−11.000	1.500		Aqueous	11.000	U	0.000
5*	Standard	Cornea	−6.700	0.520		Cornea	6.000	U	−0.300
6*	Standard	Subject eye	−7.800	−178.364	M		6.000	U	−0.500
IMA	Standard		130.000	—			94.996		0.000

When an aperture is defined on a surface, ZEMAX will display an asterisk "" symbol next to the surface number.*

Table 6.
Optical data of +5 D myopic eye by BM (image semi-diameter: 94.996 mm).

Surf: type		Comment	Radius	Thickness		Glass	Semi-diameter		Conic
*	Standard	Retina	11.000	12.880		Vitreous	8.000		0.000
1*	Standard	Lens	6.000	3.700		Lens	5.000	U	−3.000
2*	Standard		−10.000	0.100		Aqueous	5.000	U	0.000
STO	Standard	Pupil	Infinity	1.600		Aqueous	2.000	U	0.000
4	Standard		−11.000	1.500		Aqueous	11.000	U	0.000
5*	Standard	Cornea	−6.700	0.520		Cornea	6.000	U	−0.300
6*	Standard	Subject eye	−7.800	−83.003	M		6.000	U	−0.500
IMA	Standard		65.000	—			48.329		0.000

When an aperture is defined on a surface, ZEMAX will display an asterisk "" symbol next to the surface number.*

Table 7.
Optical data of +10 D myopic eye by BM (image semi-diameter: 48.329 mm).

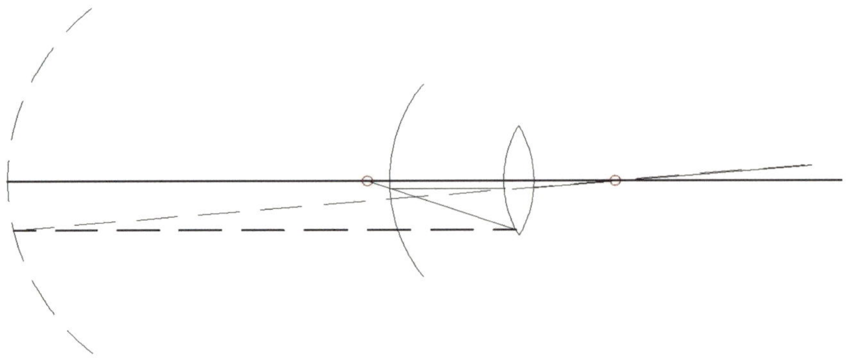

Figure 16.
Far point plane of low degree hyperopic eye by BM. It is virtual, erected, and relatively huge.

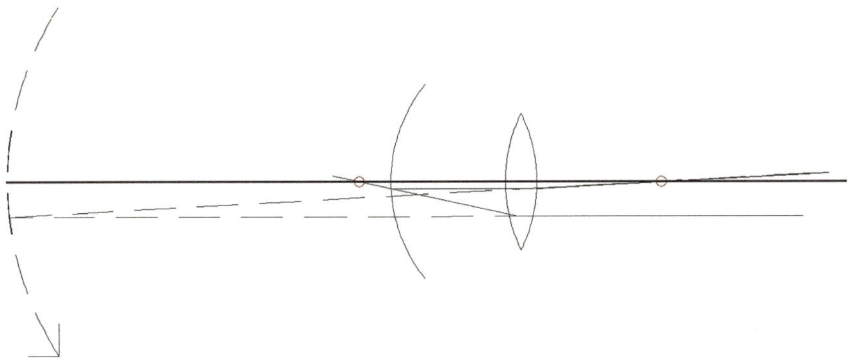

Figure 17.
Far point plane of high degree hyperopic eye by BM.

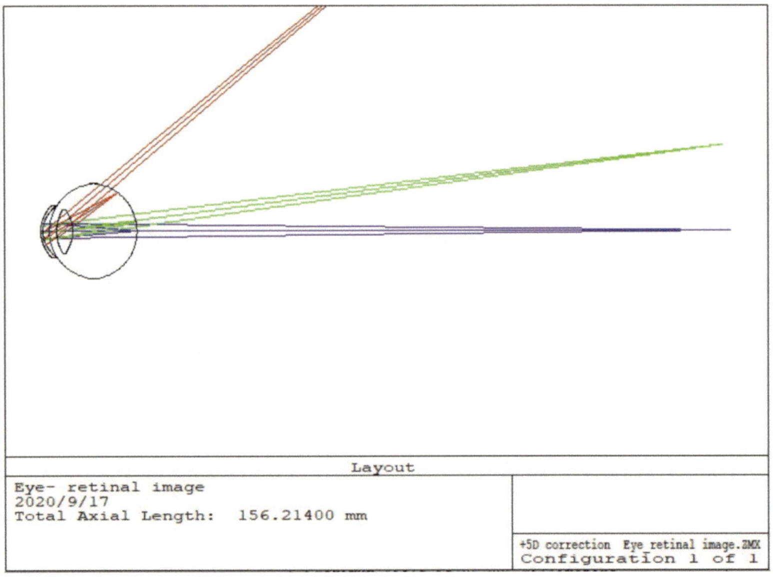

Figure 18.
Correction of +5 D hyperopia with 94.996 mm object height.

Surf: type		Comment	Radius	Thickness	Glass	Semi-diameter		Conic
*	Standard		−130.000	−156.214		0.000	U	0.000
1*	Standard	Cornea	7.800	0.520	Cornea	6.000	U	−0.500
2*	Standard		6.700	1.500	Aqueous	6.000	U	−0.300
3	Standard		11.000	1.600	Aqueous	11.000	U	0.000
*	Standard	Pupil	Infinity	0.100	Aqueous	1.500	U	0.000
5*	Standard	Lens	10.000	3.700	Lens	5.000	U	0.000
6*	Standard		−6.000	14.730	Vitreous	5.000	U	−3.250
IMA	Standard	Retina	−11.000	—	Vitreous	11.000	U	0.000

When an aperture is defined on a surface, ZEMAX will display an asterisk "" symbol next to the surface number.*

Table 8.
Optical data of +5 D hyperopia correction.

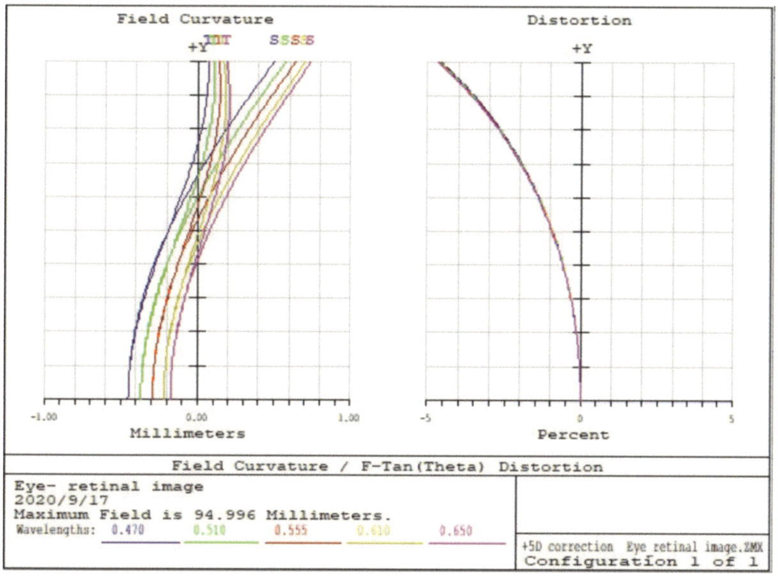

Figure 19.
Field curvature and distortion of +5 D hyperopic eye with well correction by putting the far point at the designated data from ***Table 6*** *by BM.*

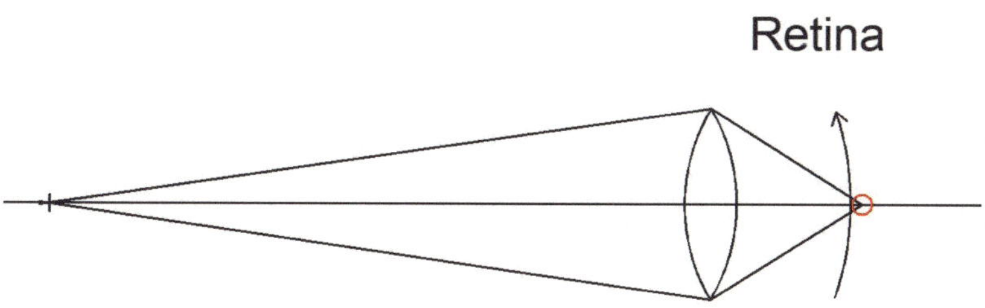

Figure 20.
Presbyopia at the distant object distance, and the image point (red dot) is assumed as the quasi focus.

Using the developed BM in Section 2 and Eq. (1), we can see how the variation of x' along with x shown in **Figures 20–22** [3] corresponding to the finite distances as the nearer object corresponding a longer focus error. The revised BM was

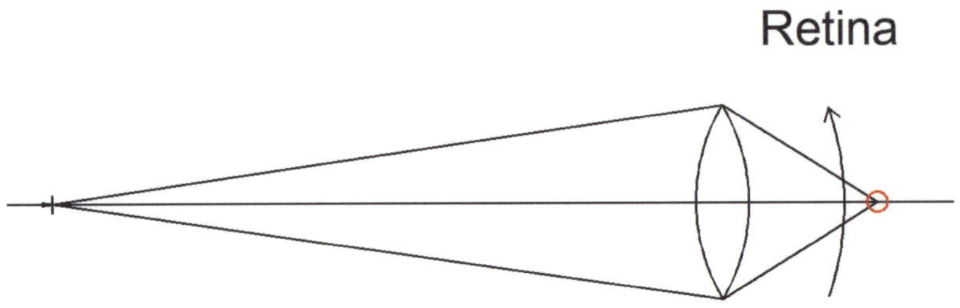

Figure 21.
Presbyopia at the intermediate object distance, and the image point (red dot) is assumed as the quasi focus.

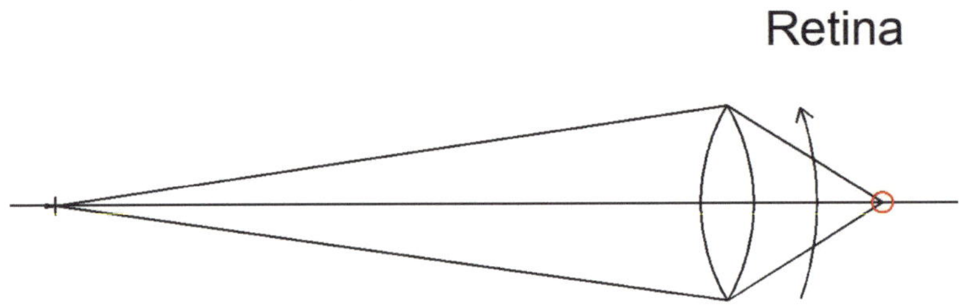

Figure 22.
Presbyopia at the near object distance, and the image point (red dot) is assumed as the quasi focus.

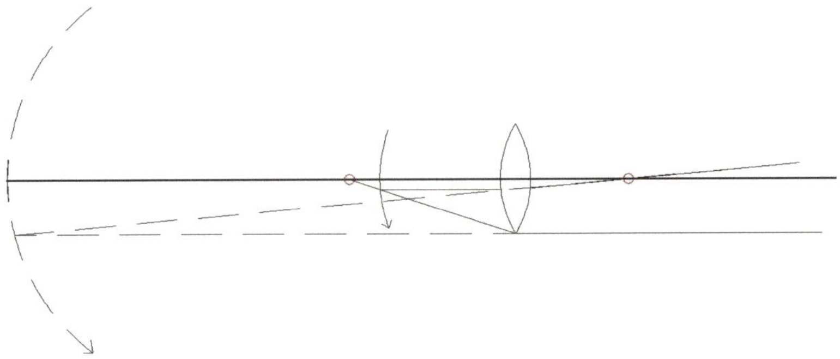

Figure 23.
Quasi far point plane of presbyopia.

introduced, and the position of the image point was assumed as the "quasi focus" of the presbyopic optics.

In presbyopic eye, by BM the quasi far point plane is located behind the retina similar with hyperopia shown in **Figure 23**. And we can see each object distance results a corresponding quasi far point plane.

Choosing the object distance as 500 mm, and setting the curvature of the eye lens with 15 mm modified from 10 mm because of the aged effect losing the accommodation of eyes power, the focus error resulted to 1.628 mm shown in **Figure 24** and **Table 9**.

By BM, the optical simulation gives much more information of the presbyopia with 1.628 mm focus error, i.e., quasi far point plan distance, image height, and curvature of the image, illustrated in **Figure 25** and **Table 10** with object height varied by 0 and 4 mm.

Then the correction of presbyopia with 1.628 mm focus error can be design by putting the quasi far point plan at the second focal point of the convex lens illustrated in **Figure 26** and **Table 11** choosing the data from **Table 10**.

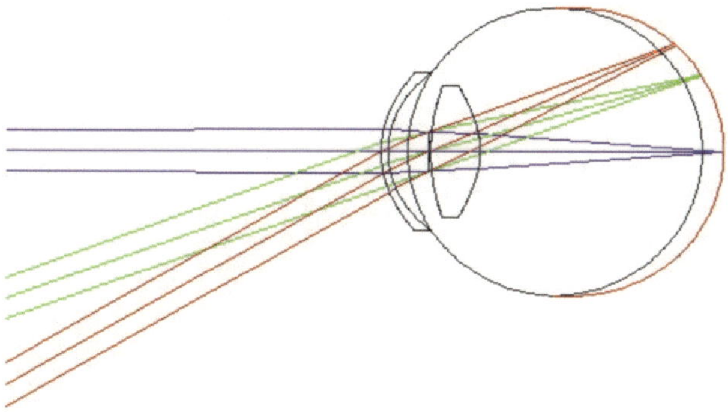

Figure 24.
Presbyopia with 1.628 mm focus error.

Surf: type		Comment	Radius	Thickness		Glass	Semi-diameter		Conic
*	Standard		Infinity	500.000			0.000	U	0.000
1*	Standard	Cornea	7.800	0.520		Cornea	6.000	U	−0.500
2*	Standard		6.700	1.500		Aqueous	6.000	U	−0.300
3	Standard		11.000	1.600		Aqueous	11.000	U	0.000
*	Standard	Pupil	Infinity	0.100		Aqueous	1.500	U	0.000
5*	Standard	Lens	15.000	3.700		Lens	5.000	U	0.000
6*	Standard		−6.000	16.580		Vitreous	5.000	U	−3.250
7	Standard		−11.000	1.628	M	Vitreous	11.000	U	0.000
IMA	Standard	Retina	−11.000	—		Vitreous	11.000	U	0.000

When an aperture is defined on a surface, ZEMAX will display an asterisk "" symbol next to the surface number.*

Table 9.
Optical data of presbyopia with 1.628 mm focus error.

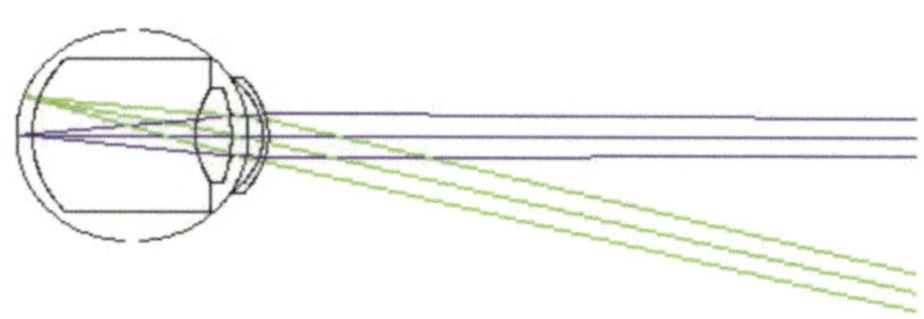

Figure 25.
Quasi far point plan of presbyopia with 1.628 mm focus error.

The image quality of correction of presbyopia of focus error with 1.628 mm is illustrated in **Figure 27** whose field curvature and distortion are well corrected.

4. Conclusion and discussion

From Sections 2 and 3, BM gives another point of view to explore the essence of image forming of eye for getting detail information of image forming of ametropia and presbyopia. And the results of optical simulation provide not only the qualitative but quantitative analyses which can be used in the design of ophthalmic lens

Surf: type		Comment	Radius	Thickness		Glass	Semi-diameter		Conic
*	Standard	Retina	11.000	1.628		Vitreous	4.000		0.000
1	Standard		11.000	16.580		Vitreous	8.000	U	0.000
2*	Standard	Lens	6.000	3.700		Lens	5.000	U	−3.000
3*	Standard		−15.000	0.100		Aqueous	5.000	U	0.000
STO	Standard	Pupil	Infinity	1.600		Aqueous	2.000	U	0.000
5	Standard		−11.000	1.500		Aqueous	11.000	U	0.000
6*	Standard	Cornea	−6.700	0.520		Cornea	6.000	U	−0.300
7*	Standard	Subject eye	−7.800	541.714	M		6.000	U	−0.500
IMA	Standard		−350.000	—			123.642		0.000

When an aperture is defined on a surface, ZEMAX will display an asterisk "" symbol next to the surface number.*

Table 10.
Optical data of presbyopia with 1.628 mm focus error.

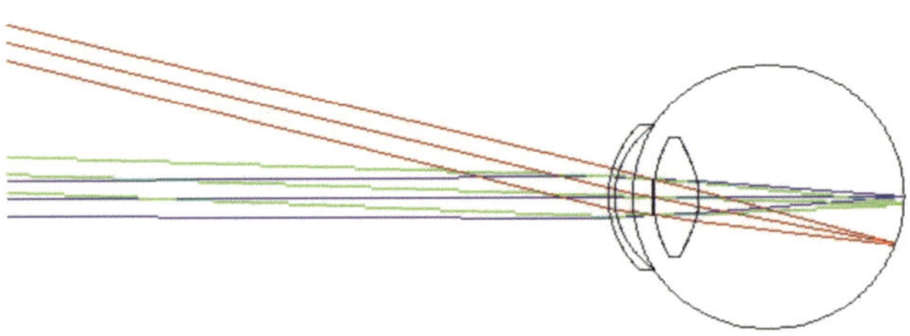

Figure 26.
Layout of correction of presbyopia with 1.628 mm focus error.

Surf: type		Radius	Thickness	Glass	Semi-diameter		Conic
*	Standard	350.000	516.086		0.000	U	0.000
1*	Standard	7.800	0.520	Cornea	6.000	U	−0.500
2*	Standard	6.700	1.500	Aqueous	6.000	U	−0.300
3	Standard	11.000	1.600	Aqueous	11.000	U	0.000
*	Standard	Infinity	0.100	Aqueous	1.500	U	0.000
5*	Standard	10.000	3.700	Lens	5.000	U	0.000
6*	Standard	−6.000	16.580	Vitreous	5.000	U	−3.250
IMA	Standard	−11.000	—	Vitreous	11.000	U	0.000

When an aperture is defined on a surface, ZEMAX will display an asterisk "" symbol next to the surface number.*

Table 11.
Optical datasheet of correction of presbyopia with 1.628 mm focus error.

such as the object distance, object height, and curvature of the object. We can also summarize the optical characteristics of ametropia listed in **Table 12**.

Similarly, the optical characteristics of presbyopic eye are listed in **Table 13**.

Applying BM, it is easy to perceive the difference between the myopia and the hyperopia. The conjugant plane of the retina formed by myopia is real and inverted, then the distance object is imaged on this conjugate plane by a concave lens to redirect the object placed on the secondary focal plane of the lens where is the far

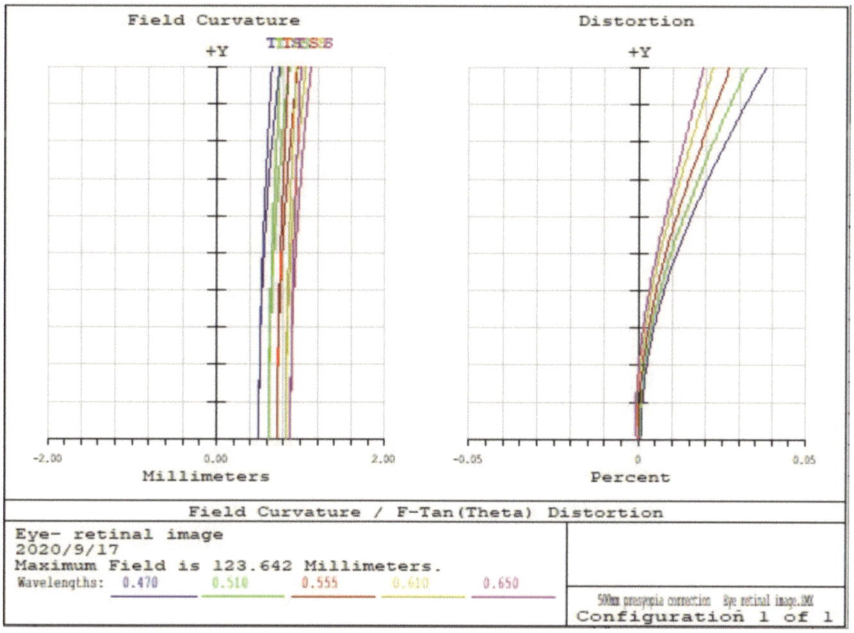

Figure 27.
Field curvature and distortion of presbyopia of focus error with 1.628 mm.

Properties / Ametropia	Retina position (object at infinity)	Position of far point plane	Type of far point plane	Type of spectacle
Myopia	Behind the focus	In front of the eye	Real, inverted	Concave lens
Hyperopia	In front of the focus	Behind the eye	Virtual, erected	Convex lens

Table 12.
Properties of ametropia.

Properties / Ametropia	Retina Position (object at infinity)	Position of far point plane	Type of far point plane	Type of spectacle
Presbyopia	In front of the quasi focus	Behind the eye	Virtual, erected	Convex PALs

Table 13.
Properties of presbyopia.

point plane of myopia. But the conjugate plane of the retina formed by hyperopia is virtual and erected, then the distance object is imaged by adding a convex lens to let the distance object lie on secondary focal plane of the lens. Eventually, either myopia or hyperopia, the image formed on the retina is inverted just like the emmetropia. And the presented chapter uses the developed BM and series graphs and tables to explain how the correction lenses fulfill these requirements by BM and optical simulation.

We can also see the object height, object curvature are critical to get a better image performance for minimizing the field of curvature and distortion either in ametropia and presbyopia. And this can be useful for ophthalmic lens manufacture to make a better fit spectacle to the glass wearer.

In conclusion, this chapter gives a rigorous analysis of image formation of eye BM. Apparently, the far point plan of ametropia and quasi far point plan of presbyopia indicate a helpful information to design a better fit spectacle concerning the object height and its shape. Suppose this will give an innovation of spectacle design. And the concept and the procedures presented in this chapter is going to be patented.

Acknowledgements

I would like to thank Asia University in Taiwan for providing a suitable research environment and supporting this research granted by No. 107-ASIA-01 and No. ASIA-108-CMUH-17.

Author details

Rung-Sheng Chen
Department of Optometry, Asia University, Taichung, Taiwan

*Address all correspondence to: rschen@asia.edu.tw

References

[1] Smith WJ. Modern Optical Engineering. 4th ed. USA: SPIE Press; 2008

[2] Atchison DA. Spectacle lens design: A review. Applied Optics. 1992;**31**(19): 3579-3585

[3] Chen R-S. Geometric analysis of ophthalmic lens by conjugate method. In: Proceedings of IEEE International Conference on Applied System Innovation. 2018. pp. 635-637

[4] Meister D. Fundamentals of progressive lens design. VisionCare Product News. 2006;**6**(9):1-6

[5] Chen R-S, Chen D-C, Chen B-Y, Hsieh S-W. Systematic design of myopic ophthalmic lens. Asian Journal of Arts and Sciences. 2010;**1**(1):83-95

[6] Smith G, Atchison DA. The Eye and Visual Optical Instruments. UK: Cambridge Press; 1997

[7] Pallikaris I, Plainis S, Charman WN. Presbyopia: Origin, Effects, and Treatments. Australia: SLACK Incorporated; 2012

[8] Sheedy JE. Prescribing Multifocal Lenses. Available from: http://www.eyecalcs.com/DWAN/pages/v1/v1c044.html